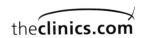
theclinics.com

# PHYSICAL MEDICINE AND REHABILITATION CLINICS OF NORTH AMERICA

## Running Injuries

GUEST EDITORS
Venu Akuthota, MD,
Mark A. Harrast, MD

CONSULTING EDITOR
George H. Kraft, MD, MS

August 2005 • Volume 16 • Number 3

**SAUNDERS**

An Imprint of Elsevier, Inc.
PHILADELPHIA   LONDON   TORONTO   MONTREAL   SYDNEY   TOKYO

**W.B. SAUNDERS COMPANY**

*A Division of Elsevier Inc.*

1600 John F. Kennedy Blvd. • Suite 1800 • Philadelphia, Pennsylvania 19103

http://www.theclinics.com

| | |
|---|---|
| **PHYSICAL MEDICINE AND REHABILITATION** | **Volume 16, Number** |
| **CLINICS OF NORTH AMERICA** | **ISSN 1047-965** |
| **August 2005** | **ISBN 1-4160-2868-** |
| Editor: Molly Jay | |

The ideas and opinions expressed in *Physical Medicine and Rehabilitation Clinics of North America* do no necessarily reflect those of the Publisher. The Publisher does not assume any responsibility for any injur and/or damage to persons or property arising out of or related to any use of the material contained i this periodical. The reader is advised to check the appropriate medical literature and the product info mation currently provided by the manufacturer of each drug to be administered to verify the dosage, th method and duration of administration, or contraindications. It is the responsibility of the treating phy sician or other health care professional, relying on independent experience and knowledge of the patien to determine drug dosages and the best treatment for the patient. Mention of any product in this issu should not be construed as endorsement by the contributors, editors, or the Publisher of the product c manufacturers' claims.

*Physical Medicine and Rehabilitation Clinics of North America* (ISSN 1047-9651) is published quarterl by W.B. Saunders Company, Corporate and Editorial Offices: 1600 John F. Kennedy Blvd., Suite 180( Philadelphia, PA 19103-2899. Accounting and Circulation Offices: 6277 Sea Harbor Drive, Orlando, F 32887-4800. Periodicals postage paid at Orlando, FL 32862, and additional mailing offices. Subscriptio price per year is $155.00 (US individuals), $238.00 (US institutions), $78.00 (US students), $188.0 (Canadian individuals), $305.00 (Canadian institutions), $108.00 (Canadian students), $215.00 (foreig individuals), $305.00 (foreign institutions), and $108.00 (foreign students). Foreign air speed deliver is included in all *Clinics* subscription prices. All prices are subject to change without notice. POSTMAS TER: Send address changes to *Physical Medicine and Rehabilitation Clinics of North America*, W.B. Saunder Company, Periodicals Fulfillment, Orlando, FL 32887-4800. **Customer Service: 1-800-654-2452 (US). Fron outside of the US, call 1-407-345-4000.**

*Physical Medicine and Rehabilitation Clinics of North America* is indexed in *Excerpta Medica, Index Medicus Cinahl*, and *Cumulative Index to Nursing and Allied Health Literature*.

Printed in the United States of America.

# CONSULTING EDITOR

**GEORGE H. KRAFT, MD, MS,** Professor, Department of Rehabilitation Medicine; Adjunct Professor of Neurology; Director, Electrodiagnostic Medicine, Western Multiple Sclerosis Center; and Co-Director, Muscular Dystrophy Clinic, The University of Washington, Seattle, Washington

# GUEST EDITORS

**VENU AKUTHOTA, MD,** Assistant Professor; Director, Residency Program and The Spine Center, University of Colorado Health Sciences Center, Denver, Colorado

**MARK A. HARRAST, MD,** Assistant Professor of Rehabilitation Medicine and Orthopaedics and Sports Medicine, Department of Rehabilitation Medicine, University of Washington, Seattle, Washington

# CONTRIBUTORS

**VENU AKUTHOTA, MD,** Assistant Professor; Director, Residency Program and The Spine Center, University of Colorado Health Sciences Center, Denver, Colorado

**KAREN P. BARR, MD,** Assistant Professor, Department of Rehabilitation Medicine, University of Washington, Seattle, Washington

**KRISHNA P. BHAT, MD,** Chief Resident, Physical Medicine and Rehabilitation Residency Program, Rush University Medical Center, Chicago, Illinois

**WALTER BROWN, MSPT, OCS,** Director of Physical Therapy, Buffalo Spine and Sports Institute, Williamsville, New York

**SHEILA A. DUGAN, MD,** Assistant Professor, Department of Physical Medicine and Rehabilitation, Rush University Medical Center, Chicao, Illinois

**MICHAEL FREDERICSON, MD,** Associate Professor, Division of Physical Medicine and Rehabilitation, Stanford University School of Medicine; Head Physician, Stanford Cross-Country and Track Teams, Stanford, California

**MICHAEL C. GERACI, JR, MD, PT,** Fellowship Program Director, Buffalo Spine and Sports Institute, Williamsville; Clinical Associate Professor, Department of Physical Medicine and Rehabilitation, State University of New York at Buffalo, Buffalo, New York; College of Osteopathic Medicine, Michigan State University, East Lansing, Michigan

**MARK A. HARRAST, MD,** Assistant Professor of Rehabilitation Medicine and Orthopaedics and Sports Medicine, Department of Rehabilitation Medicine, University of Washington, Seattle, Washington

**ANNE Z. HOCH, DO, PT,** Associate Professor, Department of Orthopaedic Surgery, Medical College of Wisconsin, Milwaukee, Wisconsin

**ALAN HRELJAC, PhD,** Associate Professor of Biomechanics, Kinesiology and Health Science Department, California State University, Sacramento, Sacramento, California

**DEYVANI HUNT, MD,** Physical Medicine and Rehabilitation, Department of Orthopaedic Surgery, Washington University School of Medicine, St. Louis, Missouri

**PAUL H. LENTO, MD,** Attending Physician, Rehabilitation Institute of Chicago Spine, Sports, and Rehabilitation Center; Assistant Professor, Department of Physical Medicine and Rehabilitation, Northwestern University Feinberg School of Medicine, Chicago, Illinois

**TAMMARA MOORE, PT,** Founder, Sports and Orthopedic Leaders Physical Therapy, Oakland; Consultant, University of California, Berkeley Athletic Teams, Berkeley, California

**MICHELLE PEPPER, MD,** Medical College of Wisconsin, Milwaukee, Wisconsin

**CHRISTOPHER T. PLASTARAS, MD,** Attending Physician, Rehabilitation Institute of Chicago, Spine and Sports Rehabilitation Center; Assistant Professor, Department of Physical Medicine and Rehabilitation, Northwestern University Feinberg School of Medicine, Chicago, Illinois

**HEIDI PRATHER, DO,** Chief of Section, Physical Medicine and Rehabilitation, Department of Orthopaedic Surgery, Washington University School of Medicine, St. Louis, Missouri

**JOEL PRESS, MD,** Medical Director, Rehabilitation Institute of Chicago, Spine and Sports Rehabilitation Center; Associate Professor, Department of Physical Medicine and Rehabilitation, Northwestern University Feinberg School of Medicine, Chicago, Illinois

**JOSHUA D. RITTENBERG, MD,** Attending Physician, Rehabilitation Institute of Chicago, Spine and Sports Rehabilitation Center; Assistant Professor, Department of Physical Medicine and Rehabilitation, Northwestern University Feinberg School of Medicine, Chicago, Illinois

**KATHRYN E. RITTENBERG, DPT,** Staff Physical Therapist, Rehabilitation Institute of Chicago, Spine and Sports Rehabilitation Center, Chicago, Illinois

**WILLIAM J. SULLIVAN, MD,** Attending Physician, University of Colorado Health Sciences Center, The Spine Center at University Hospital; Assistant Professor, Department of Physical Medicine and Rehabilitation, University of Colorado School of Medicine, Denver, Colorado

**MICHAEL H. YAMASHITA, PT,** Partner, Eastside Sports Rehab, Kirkland, Washington

# CONTENTS

> A thorough understanding of proper running biomechanics will al-
> low the clinician to prevent and treat running injuries. This article
> details the anatomy and biomechanics of the lower limb as the
> body moves through the running gait cycle. Factors that distin-
> guish running from walking are described and the effect of velocity
> on running economy is discussed. Functional biomechanics of run-
> ning gait are discussed, which explains the concepts of pronation
> and supination. The authors also explain various methods of run-
> ning gait analysis and their relevance to the understanding of run-
> ning biomechanics.

> In most cases, a detailed history provides the information that is
> necessary for the clinician to diagnose the injured runner correctly.
> To treat the injury and guide a successful rehabilitation program,
> the physical examination must go beyond the standard regional
> musculoskeletal examination. The victims (tissue injury) and the
> culprits (biomechanical deficits) must be identified to facilitate
> treatment. Gait and other dynamic assessments help to reveal un-
> derlying deficits in function that may have contributed to injury. In
> short, the entire functional kinetic chain must be considered and
> weak links identified.

includes a brief review of temperature regulation during exercise as it relates to hyperthermia and hypothermia. Finally, the last section covers the metabolic conditions that typically are encountered in a runner who requires medical attention, including several myths and controversies regarding fluid replacement and the causes of exercise-associated hyponatremia.

## FORTHCOMING ISSUES

## RECENT ISSUES

Phys Med Rehabil Clin N Am
16 (2005) xi–xii

PHYSICAL MEDICINE
AND REHABILITATION
CLINICS OF
NORTH AMERICA

Foreword

# Running Injuries

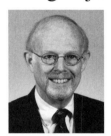

George H. Kraft, MD, MS
*Consulting Editor*

Give about two [hours], every day, to exercise; for health must not be
sacrificed to learning. A strong body makes the mind strong.
— *Thomas Jefferson, letter to Peter Carr, 19 August 1785*

Many healthy people are now taking Jefferson's admonition to heart; it
seems everyone is running for health. Sometimes it is out of doors,
sometimes on an inside track, and sometimes on a treadmill. People are
running around the neighborhood, and they are running at the health club.
Running has become a national pastime.

And for good reason. Running may be the perfect aerobic exercise. It
gives the benefits of aerobic activity, and it can be done with virtually no
equipment or cost. But running has its downside, too. Done improperly, and
with inadequate shoes, it can cause injuries. Even persons who do everything
right can sustain injuries. The fact that it is typically done several times
a week only increases the chance of injury. And that is what this issue of the
*Physical Medicine and Rehabilitation Clinics of North America* is about.

Musculoskeletal and sports medicine have become arguably the most
popular part of the field of physical medicine and rehabilitation. Year after
year, many of our graduating fourth-year residents enroll in sports and
spine fellowships. There is demand for their services in all parts of the
United States.

As a reflection of this trend in the field, the *Clinics* series is publishing
more and more issues on musculoskeletal medicine. This issue on running

doi:10.1016/j.pmr.2005.03.003

injuries continues this trend. It is a pleasure to once again work with
Dr. Mark Harrast and to welcome Dr. Venu Akuthnota to this series.
Together, they have created an issue of practical information on prevention
and treatment of injuries to the runner.

The fundamentals—biomechanics and functional assessment—are discussed first. Following this, prevention of overuse and injuries of the three
regions of the lower limb (ie, the hip, knee, and foot) are thoroughly
discussed. The female runner has unique concerns, and they are examined as
well. Next, the platform making running possible—the shoe—is presented.
Finally, the downed runner is discussed.

I am convinced that you, the reader, will find the information presented
in this issue to be of practical value in treating your patients. As the guest
editors have pointed out in their preface: "This issue can be used as a clinical
reference tool for many of our patients with lower limb (a more accurate
term than "extremity"—technically, the extreme portion [ankle and foot]
of the limb) complaints." This is the intent.

Let me end this foreword with an invitation to the reader to contact me
with your thoughts on this series. Are we fulfilling your needs? Do you have
any topics you want to see presented? And are you interested in being
a guest editor? Please let me know.

George H. Kraft, MD, MS
*Department of Rehabilitation Medicine*
*University of Washington School of Medicine*
*1959 NE Pacific Street, Box 356490*
*Seattle, WA 98195-6490, USA*

*E-mail address:* ghkraft@u.washington.edu

ELSEVIER
SAUNDERS

Phys Med Rehabil Clin N Am
16 (2005) xiii–xiv

PHYSICAL MEDICINE
AND REHABILITATION
CLINICS OF
NORTH AMERICA

## Preface

# Running Injuries

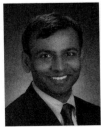 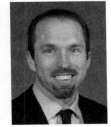

Venu Akuthota, MD       Mark A. Harrast, MD
*Guest Editors*

It is our sincere honor and privilege to put together this compendium on running injuries. Although many articles and one major text have been devoted to running injuries, we wanted to present an approach with an emphasis on physiatry—that is, the incorporation of function into evaluation and treatment. This "function thing" sounds (and is) elemental, but all of us need to be reminded that we can always be more functional. Incorporating a functional and thus less regional approach to the rehabilitation of musculoskeletal injuries is a change for the better. This is fitting for our practice as physiatrists, because we are the ideal champions of function. As such, we hope this issue of the *Physical Medicine and Rehabilitation Clinics of North America* demonstrates our role in treating running injuries.

As you read this issue, you will realize that the lower limb injuries that the authors present and the evidence-based management strategies offered are not all necessarily unique to the runner. This issue can be used as a clinical reference tool for many patients who have lower limb complaints, and we hope it will also be very useful and generalizable for musculoskeletal practice.

To that end, we have gathered a group of experts in the field of sports medicine. To be true to the multidisciplinary spirit of physical medicine and rehabilitation, we have included physiatrists, physical therapists, an exercise physiologist, and a kinesiologist, spanning clinicians and scientists. Sadly, near the completion of this issue, we learned that Dr. Scott Nadler, one of

1047-9651/05/$ - see front matter © 2005 Elsevier Inc. All rights reserved.
doi:10.1016/j.pmr.2005.05.001

*pmr.theclinics.com*

the prospective contributing authors, passed away. He was a true inspiration and role model for physiatrists wanting to expand the field through education and research. His research serves as the basis for the kinetic chain concept that is so important in the treatment of running injuries. We dedicate this issue to a true hero, father, husband, and friend: Scott Nadler.

Venu Akuthota, MD
*Department of Physical Medicine and Rehabilitation*
*University of Colorado School of Medicine*
*PO Box 6510, Mail Stop F712*
*Aurora, CO 80045, USA*

*E-mail address:* venu.akuthota@uchsc.edu

Mark A. Harrast, MD
*Department of Rehabilitation Medicine*
*University of Washington*
*1959 NE Pacific Street, Box 356490*
*Seattle, WA 98195, USA*

*E-mail address:* mharrast@u.washington.edu

ELSEVIER
SAUNDERS

Phys Med Rehabil Clin N Am
16 (2005) 603–621

PHYSICAL MEDICINE
AND REHABILITATION
CLINICS OF
NORTH AMERICA

# Biomechanics and Analysis
# of Running Gait

## Sheila A. Dugan, MD*, Krishna P. Bhat, MD

*Department of Physical Medicine and Rehabilitation, Rush University Medical Center,
1725 West Harrison, Suite 970, Chicago, IL 60614, USA*

The increased awareness of aerobic exercise to maintain a healthy lifestyle has made jogging and running more popular than ever. As the number of people that is engaged in these activities grows, increased incidences of acute and chronic running injuries naturally occur. To prevent and properly treat these injuries, a thorough understanding of normal walking and running gait is critical.

Proper running biomechanics involves synchronous movements of all of the components of the kinetic chain. The foot serves as the link between the ambulatory surface and the remainder of this chain. The foot's many functions include adaptation to uneven terrain, proprioception for proper position and balance, and leverage for propulsion. During the gait cycle, foot motion facilitates, and can be affected by, compensatory movement of the other bones and joints in the lower extremity. Improper alignment from the lumbar spine and lower limb below can alter mechanics and lead to injury. Therefore, it is essential to understand the biomechanics of running gait along the entire kinetic chain.

This article describes the anatomy of the foot and its relation to the gait cycle, discusses similarities and differences between walking and running gait, explains the contributions of the muscles and joints intrinsic and extrinsic to the foot, and demonstrates the effect of velocity on the economy of gait. The concepts of pronation and supination are discussed in detail. Running biomechanics of lower limb joints and muscles are described in all three cardinal planes (sagittal, frontal, and transverse). Also, the use of various methods of gait analysis are described along with their relevance to particular constituents of the running gait cycle. A thorough understanding of running gait allows a treating physician to recognize different

* Corresponding author.
*E-mail address:* sheila_dugan@rush.edu (S.A. Dugan).

mechanisms of injury and allows proper treatment and prevention of running injuries.

### Anatomy and biomechanics

Running biomechanics are dictated by lower limb anatomy, particularly the joints of the foot and ankle. The axis of rotation with each joint allows for joints to have a predominant plane of motion, perpendicular to that axis. For example, the talocrural joint's anatomy allows for an axis of rotation that mostly is in the frontal plane (Fig. 1). Consequently, the talocrural joint has its predominant range of motion in the sagittal plane. Each joint moves in all planes with a predominant plane of motion. So-called "pronation" and "supination" are triplanar movements that involve multiple joints of the foot and ankle (Box 1). Pronation and supination of the foot and ankle causes obligate motion in the entire lower limb kinetic chain (Table 1).

The true ankle joint, also termed the talocrural joint, incorporates the articulation between the surface of the tibia and fibula with the superior surface of the talus. This joint primarily moves in the sagittal plane and allows dorsiflexion and plantarflexion. Because the lateral malleolus is located posterior relative to the medial malleolus, the talocrural joint axis travels primarily in the frontal plane with some posterior orientation from

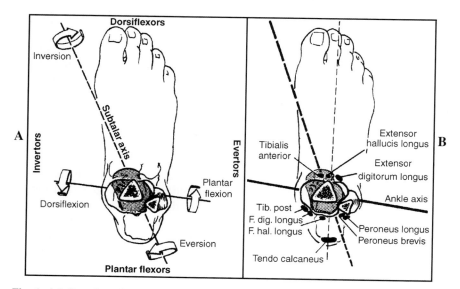

Fig. 1. (*A*) Rotation about the ankle and subtalar joint axes. (*B*) Musculotendinous unit position in relation to the ankle and subtalar joint axes. Tib post, tibialis posterior; F. dig, flexor digitorum; F. hal, flexor hallucis. (*From* Mann RA, Mann JA. Biomechanics of the foot. In: Goldberg B, Hsu JD, editors. Atlas of orthoses and assistive devices. 3rd edition. St. Louis (MO): Mosby; 1997. p. 145; with permission.)

---

**Box 1. Multiplanar motions of pronation and supination in the foot and ankle in weight bearing**

*Pronation*
Ankle dorsiflexion
Subtalar eversion
Forefoot abduction

*Supination*
Ankle plantarflexion
Subtalar inversion
Forefoot adduction

---

(Nonweight-bearing pronation = ankle plantarflexion, talus internal rotation, and talus adduction)

---

the medial to lateral side. Functionally, this results in talocrural joint movement in the transverse plane and little movement in the frontal plane. In the open kinetic chain, as dorsiflexion occurs, there is accompanying external rotation of the tibia. In the closed kinetic chain, as with the stance phase of ambulation, dorsiflexion causes pronation of the foot with internal rotation of the tibia [1]. The average range of motion in the ankle joint is approximately 45°, with up to 20° of dorsiflexion and 25° to 35° of plantarflexion [2].

Table 1
Effects of pronation and supination up the kinetic chain

|  | Pronation | | | Supination | | |
|---|---|---|---|---|---|---|
|  | Sagittal | Frontal | Transverse | Sagittal | Frontal | Transverse |
| Lumbosacral | Extension | Lat flexion same side | Protraction | Extension | Lat flexion opp side | Retraction |
| Pelvis | Anterior rotation | Translation and elevation, same side | Forward rot same side | Anterior rotation | Translation opp side; depression same side | Rear rot same side |
| Hip | Flexion | Adduction | Internal rotation | Extension | Abduction | External rotation |
| Knee | Flexion | Abduction | Internal rotation | Extension | Adduction | External rotation |
| Ankle | PF-DF |  | Internal rotation | DF-PF |  | External rotation |
| STJ | PF | Eversion | Adduction | DF | Inversion | Abduction |
| MTJ | DF | Inversion | Abduction | PF | Eversion | Adduction |

*Abbreviations:* DF, dorsiflexion; Lat, lateral; MTJ, midtalar joint; Opp, opposite; PF, plantarflexion; rot, rotation; STJ, subtalar joint.

The subtalar joint (STJ), between the talus and calcaneus, consists of three articular facets—anterior, middle, and posterior. These separate articulations function as a single joint and allow the complex triplanar motions of pronation and supination. The axis of this joint runs downward, posteriorly in the sagittal plane and laterally in the transverse plane (see Fig. 1; Fig. 2). In the transverse plane, the joint axis is oriented approximately 23° medial to the long axis of the foot [3]. Interindividual variation in orientation does occur, with a range of 4° to 47° (see Fig. 2A). In the sagittal plane, the joint axis is oriented, on average, 41° relative to the sole of the foot and runs posteriorly and distally from the dorsal aspect of the neck of the talus to the posterolateral corner of the calcaneus [3]. Interindividual variation ranges from 21° to 69° (see Fig. 2B). As the joint axis becomes more horizontal, such as with a flat foot, eversion and inversion occur to a greater extent than abduction and adduction. Also, as the axis gets closer to the sagittal plane, less dorsiflexion and plantarflexion is allowed [4]. The STJ is analogous to an oblique hinge because of its configuration in relation to the remainder of the foot [5]. This allows the foot to move in a complex, but predictable, manner.

Pronation is defined classically as abduction and eversion of the foot along with hindfoot eversion. Supination is described classically as adduction and inversion of the foot along with hindfoot inversion; however, pronation and supination will cause multiple, multiplanar proximal joint movement. The orientation of the STJ relative to the tibia also results in a mitered hinge effect. Torque that is developed by movement of the foot is transmitted proximally and results in internal or external rotation of the tibia [1]. In weight bearing,

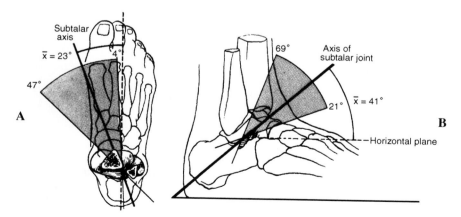

Fig. 2. Subtalar joint axis within the foot. (*A*) Transverse plane. (*B*) Sagittal plane. $\bar{X}$, average angle of joint axis. (*From* Mann RA, Mann JA. Biomechanics of the foot. In: Goldberg B, Hsu JD, editors. Atlas of orthoses and assistive devices. 3rd edition. St. Louis (MO): Mosby; 1997. p. 139; with permission.)

there is a 1:1 relationship between the degree of supination relative to tibial external rotation and pronation relative to tibial internal rotation [6].

The STJ has several functions during normal ambulation. Control of plantar surface pressure and contact with the ground is dictated by motion at the STJ. Stress dampening on the heel occurs during gait as forces are transmitted through the STJ to the midfoot and forefoot. Also, triplanar motion about this joint axis results in either a flexible or rigid foot during progression of gait (see later discussion).

STJ or calcaneal eversion, caused by ground reaction forces after foot strike, precipitates a cascade of events in the rest of the foot. The midfoot joints, namely the calcaneocuboid and talonavicular joints, allow eversion/abduction and inversion/adduction of the forefoot. The midfoot joints, also collectively termed the transverse tarsal joint, have longitudinal axes that are similar to the STJ. Thus, these pair of joints also have been dubbed as the secondary STJ. Their oblique axes are close to that of the talocrural joint and provide mainly plantarflexion and dorsiflexion. When the hindfoot everts, the axes of these two separate joint components become parallel, and allow for pronation and increased motion within this two-joint complex. With hindfoot inversion, supination occurs and the joint axes converge, which causes this joint complex to "lock" into a rigid configuration [7]. This concept is important to consider as the foot progresses through the stance phase from initial contact to terminal stance. In essence, pronation necessitates a flexible foot for shock absorption, whereas supination necessitates a rigid foot for propulsion.

The tarsometatarsal (TMT) joints can be divided into five rays. The first ray is composed of the medial cuneiform and the first metatarsal. Motion allowed at this joint is primarily a combination of dorsiflexion/inversion/adduction and plantarflexion/eversion/abduction [5]. The second ray contains the intermediate cuneiform and second metatarsal. The second metatarsal is recessed and firmly mortised into the base of the first and third metatarsal–cuneiform joints. This bone is subjected to high stress as a result of the inherent stability as the foot progresses through the stance phase in preparation for propulsion [5]. The lateral cuneiform and third metatarsal along with the fourth metatarsal make up the third and fourth rays. Motion at these rays is limited primarily to plantarflexion and dorsiflexion. The fifth ray (fifth metatarsal) allows some pronation and supination in relation to the cuboid.

The metatarsal break is an important phenomenon that is created by the metatarsophalangeal joints. These joints extend about an oblique joint axis that extends from the head of the second metatarsal to the head of the fifth metatarsal [5]. Motion at this joint predominantly is flexion and extension. As the foot progresses through the stance phase just before toe-off, this axis allows the foot to become rigid as this joint is extending [8]. This supination results in an ideal rigid platform for efficient propulsion as the leg prepares to advance through the swing phase.

The anatomic uniqueness of the plantar fascia also helps to create the solid structural platform that is needed for propulsion. It originates from the medial tubercle of the calcaneus and inserts around the metatarsal heads to the base of the proximal phalanges. It crosses the transverse tarsal and metatarsophalangeal joints and serves as a passive restraint. At the metatarsophalangeal attachment, the Spanish windlass mechanism is formed (Fig. 3). As extension occurs at the metatarsophalangeal joint just before toe-off, the plantar fascia tightens and pulls the calcaneus and metatarsal heads together [9]. This heightens the longitudinal arch of the foot and forces the transverse tarsal joint into a forced flexion position, and thereby, creates a solid structural support. In addition, the intrinsic foot muscles actively contract to provide further stability of the foot.

The ligaments within the foot also provide passive stability. Ligaments, along with muscular support and the unique bone architecture of the foot, form two longitudinal arches (medial and lateral) and a transverse arch. The medial foot ligaments are thicker than the lateral ligaments. This design prevents hyperpronation during ambulation. The arches of the foot create weight-bearing points, primarily on the calcaneus and the metatarsal heads. The sesamoid bones decrease force on the plantar surface of the first metatarsal head just before toe-off. The unique configuration of these arches allows the foot to be mobile to adjust to the ground surface and rigid in preparation to push off the ground for the sake of propulsion.

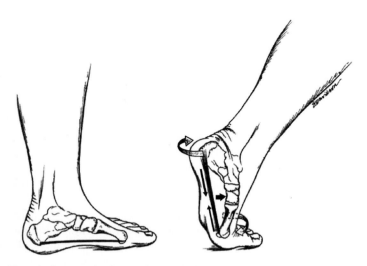

Fig. 3. The windlass mechanism. After heel-off, metatarsophalangeal extension increases tension on the plantar fascia (*converging arrows*). The transverse tarsal joint is forced into flexion (*arrowhead*), which increases stability as the foot prepares to push off. (*From* Geiringer SR. Biomechanics of the running foot and related injuries. Phys Med Rehabil State Art Rev 1997;11(3):569–82; with permission.)

The muscles of the lower leg and foot work in an eccentric and concentric fashion. Eccentric work is muscle contraction while fibers are lengthening; concentric work is muscle contraction while fibers are shortening. With running, the greatest amount of muscle work is done in an eccentric fashion. The pronation phase of gait involves mostly eccentric contraction to provide for joint control and shock absorption. The supination phase of gait involves mostly concentric contraction of various muscles, particularly the gluteals, to provide for acceleration and propulsion.

Although muscles can work in all three planes, muscle fiber orientation often dictates a preferred plane. For instance, the gluteus maximus has muscle fibers that are oriented in an oblique (transverse) fashion; therefore, this powerful muscle becomes an ideal leg external rotator (by way of concentric contraction) and controls leg internal rotation (by way of eccentric contraction). Another key muscle in running is the gastrosoleus complex, commonly considered to be a pure plantarflexor. Yet, this complex also contributes to the transverse plane motion of hindfoot inversion because of its location in relation to the STJ axis [8]. This allows the gastrocnemius-soleus to contribute to supination as the foot progresses through the gait cycle.

## Walking versus running

Running, like walking, is a series of pronations and supinations. Running is distinguished from walking by increased velocity, or distance traveled per unit time, and the presence of an airborne or float phase (Box 2). Judges in race walking determine that participants are running illegally if they observe a period of time when both feet are off the ground. During a running gait cycle, there are two periods of float when neither foot is in contact with the ground (Fig. 4). This results in decreased time in stance phase and increased

---

**Box 2. Differences between running and walking**

Increased velocity
Increased ground reaction forces
Float phase
No double stance phase
Decreased stance phase and increased swing phase
Overlap of swing phase rather than stance phase
Requires more range of motion of all lower limb joints
Requires greater eccentric muscle contraction
Initial contact varies, depending on speed
Decreased center of gravity with increased speed
Decreased base of support

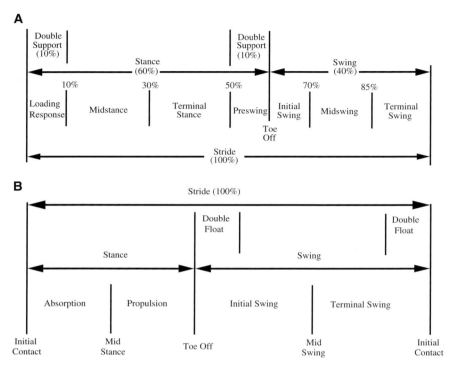

Fig. 4. Gait cycle with phases and individual components. (*A*) Walking. (*B*) Running. (*From* Ounpuu S. The biomechanics of walking and running. Clin Sport Med 1994;13(4):843–63; with permission.)

time in swing phase. As velocity continues to increase, further reduction in stance phase occurs, whereas swing phase duration increases. Unlike walking, the forward momentum that is needed for running is produced by the swinging leg and arms, rather than the stance leg [10].

Runners also require more from their joints and muscles than walkers. A greater joint excursion has been noted with hip flexion, knee flexion, and ankle dorsiflexion with running [11]. Other joints also likely go through a greater range of motion with running, such as the joints of the lumbar spine and pelvis. Increasing speed of running increases the amount of joint excursion, particularly in the sagittal plane [11]. Some investigators empirically noted a greater degree of transverse plane motion with sprinting. To control this motion, greater eccentric work is required from the muscles of the lower leg.

*Changes in running gait with increased velocity*

Running can be classified by speed. Jogging, or submaximal running, can be defined as velocity from 5 mph to 10 mph, whereas sprinting occurs at speeds of greater than 10 mph [6]. Characteristic changes in gait occur as velocity increases. As with walking, the center of gravity of the body shifts during running in a sinusoidal curve in space; however, during running, the body maintains a forward lean throughout the gait cycle. The line of progression from step to step is at or near the midline to minimize lateral shift in center of gravity. As speed is increased, the lower extremity joints increase their range of motion to decrease the vertical shift in center of gravity [3,12]. Thus, faster runners require more flexibility and eccentric muscle strength than slower runners.

Speed and length of gait can be described using the terms: cadence, stride length, and step length. Cadence is equal to the number of steps per unit time (usually steps/min). Stride length is the distance between successive initial contacts of the same foot. Step length is the distance from initial contact of one foot to initial contact of the opposite foot. Temporal and spatial variables during running generally are interrelated. Velocity increase is achieved by increasing step lengths followed by increasing cadence [11]. With elevation in velocity, there is more time spent in float phase. Stride and step lengths are a function of leg length and total height and coincide with the ability to increase these lengths while velocity increases [11].

As running velocity increases, the point of initial contact can change. During submaximal running, the lateral heel typically contacts the ground first, whereas in sprinting, the midfoot makes initial contact [3]. This places the foot in slight plantarflexion at impact [13]. Dorsiflexion still occurs directly after initial contact as during submaximal running, but the heel does not touch the ground during sprinting [3]. The remainder of stance phase mimics submaximal running, except for increased joint range of motion. During the terminal portion of swing phase, the foot begins to plantarflex during sprinting so that the midfoot can contact the ground [5].

Total gait cycle duration, as well as stance phase duration in relation to swing phase, diminishes as velocity of running increases. This results in increased velocity of lower extremity range of motion as events of the gait cycle need to occur within a shorter period of time [6]. The higher eccentric contractions that occur to control joint motion will result in higher energy expenditure. The increased range of motion in the lower extremity also serves to minimize vertical displacement of the body center of gravity [12]. The end result is increased energy cost as velocity increases to a sprint, which therefore limits the absolute running distance.

As velocity increases, running efficiency or economy changes. Running economy was traditionally measured by assessing oxygen use at a given velocity [14]. The energy cost of running is not only determined by speed but also by running biomechanics. An ideal model for economic running has yet to be found. Numerous factors, which are beyond the scope of this chapter, may affect running efficiency. For a particular individual, training allows the body to biomechanically adapt over time to achieve the least energy-expending pattern of running gait.

**Gait cycle**

The gait cycle is the period from initial contact of one foot to the next initial contact of the same foot. In normal walking, there are two phases of gait – stance and swing. During one gait cycle in walking, stance phase represents 60% of the cycle while swing phase represents the remaining 40% (Fig. 4). Double support, when two limbs are in contact with ground, occurs during the first and last 10% of a particular stance phase. Single limb support is equal to the swing time of the opposite limb.

The running gait cycle can be divided into stance phase, swing phase, and float phase. The first half of the stance phase is concerned with force absorption (pronation), whereas the second half is responsible for propulsion (supination). In Fig. 4B, stance phase is divided into subphases of initial contact to midstance, and midstance to toe-off. To understand the biomechanical events during running, stance phase can be divided into three major components: (1) initial contact to foot flat, (2) foot flat to heel-off, and (3) heel-off to toe-off [1]. Swing phase during running can be divided into initial swing and terminal swing; float phase occurs at the beginning of initial swing and the end of terminal swing.

*Initial contact to foot flat*

At initial contact during running, the lateral heel contacts the ground with the foot in a slightly supinated position [3,15]. This occurs as the leg swings toward the line of progression in midline, with the leg in a functional varus of 8° to 14° at this point. The calcaneus is inverted approximately 4° at initial contact in an average runner [12,16]. During walking, the ankle is plantarflexed, on average, 8° at heel strike and continues to 14° as the remainder of the foot contacts the ground [17]. In running, there is no plantarflexion after heel strike as the foot actually progresses into dorsiflexion [18]. This lack of plantarflexion in running causes increased pronation, but less supination. The tibialis anterior acts eccentrically during walking to cause a smooth plantarflexion, and contracts concentrically during running to stabilize the ankle and possibly to accelerate the tibia over the fixed foot as a mechanism to maintain and increase velocity [3,19]. At the same time, the gastrocnemius-soleus contracts eccentrically to control forward tibial progression and provide stability to the ankle [3].

Energy absorption or weight acceptance is a key function of the lower extremity during this phase of running gait. Vertical ground reaction force may reach a magnitude of 2.2 times body weight after heel contact in running compared with 1.1 times body weight during walking [10,20,21]. Factors that allow proper impact absorption are joint motion, eccentric muscle contraction, and articular cartilage compression [22]. Along with dorsiflexion at the ankle joint, hip and knee flexion help to dissipate the force of impact at heel contact [3].

STJ pronation is another major mechanism of shock absorption. As forward progression occurs, the STJ pronates within the first 20% of the stance phase to allow solid contact of the foot with the ground [23]. AS a result of the mitered hinge effect, pronation is accompanied by hindfoot eversion and tibial internal rotation. Pronation allows the transverse tarsal joint axes to become parallel, and increases mobility at this joint and in the forefoot. The foot can accommodate to uneven terrain and dissipate energy as it conforms to the ground surface.

Eccentric contraction of the rectus femoris after initial contact controls the height of the body center of gravity and resists excess knee flexion as the line of ground reaction force passes posterior to the knee joint. The hamstrings, which act as hip extensors, are active throughout the stance phase as the body progresses forward on the fixed limb [11]. Stability of the lower extremity at initial contact is provided by the hip adductors [24]. The adductors remain active throughout the running cycle as opposed to walking, when they are active only from swing phase to the middle of stance phase [25].

## Foot flat to heel-off

As forward progression continues through the middle of stance phase, dorsiflexion increases to a maximum of 20° in running as compared with 14° during walking [16,26,27]. During this portion of gait the foot is fixed to the ground; therefore, dorsiflexion occurs as a result of the forward progression of the tibia. Maximum dorsiflexion occurs when the body center of gravity already has passed anterior to the base of support. Just before this, maximum pronation occurs, approximately when the body center of gravity has passed anterior to the base of support [23]. At maximum pronation, the transverse tarsal joint axes are parallel, and allow increased mobility and forefoot accommodation to the underfoot surface [10,28]. The point of maximum pronation also marks the end of the absorptive component of stance phase; the subsequent propulsion component occurs through the remainder of the stance phase.

Control of pronation is provided by eccentric contraction of the tibialis posterior and gastrocnemius-soleus complex [29,30]. Forward progression of the tibia is controlled by the gastrocnemius-soleus. As ground reaction force travels anteriorly through the knee joint, cocontraction of the quadriceps and hamstring stabilizes the knee joint.

After maximum pronation, supination at the STJ begins [5]. As the opposite limb swings forward, pelvic rotation occurs and results in an external rotation torque of the stance limb. The external rotation of the tibia causes inversion at the calcaneus with subsequent supination of the foot. Initiation of supination marks the end of this phase as the heel begins to rise off the ground.

*Heel-off to toe-off*

Continued forward progression of the opposite limb and body prepares the stance limb to initiate propulsion. Ankle plantarflexion under concentric contraction of the gastrocnemius-soleus serves a few important functions at this point in the running gait. Acceleration of the stance limb as it prepares for propulsion is initiated by plantarflexion [24]. Also, as plantarflexion occurs while the forefoot is fixed to the ground, the stance phase limb is lengthened, and thus, minimizes the decrease in center of gravity as the opposite limb swings forward and prepares to contact the ground [28,31]. Lastly, plantarflexion contributes to increased contralateral stride length, and enhances the efficiency of running [8].

Supination of the foot starts at heel-off and continues for the remainder of the stance phase. Supination causes convergence of the transverse tarsal joint axes and results in a rigid foot configuration. Several important factors allow this to occur and provide increased stability of the foot as it prepares to push off the ground powerfully and efficiently to propel the limb forward [8]. External rotation of the stance limb causes STJ supination as a result of the mitered hinge effect. Gastrocnemius-soleus contraction causes hindfoot inversion and leads to STJ supination. The metatarsal break phenomenon contributes to supination as extension occurs at the metatarsophalangeal joint. This joint extension also leads to increased tension of the plantar fascia, which provides stability to the transverse tarsal joint through the Spanish windlass mechanism. Finally, the intrinsic foot muscles (in particular the abductor hallucis, flexor hallucis brevis, abductor digiti minimi, and flexor digiti minimi brevis), which cross the transverse tarsal joint, contract and stabilize this joint in a similar fashion to the plantar fascia [8].

During this portion of stance phase, maximum ground reaction force occurs as the foot pushes off the ground and thrusts the body forward. The magnitude of vertical ground reaction force may reach 2.8 times body weight with running compared with 1.3 times body weight in walking [20,21]. Each of the factors that contribute to the formation of a rigid foot is crucial to generate the force that is required at this instant of running gait.

At the termination of stance phase, the gastrocnemius-soleus stops functioning and contraction of the anterior tibialis begins. As the foot prepares to leave the ground, knee and hip extension is needed to add to the thrust of the body as it progresses into the initial float phase. Neither the hip nor the knee extends beyond neutral with running, even at toe-off [27]. The hamstrings convert from a stabilizing flexor of the knee to an active extensor of the hip [6]. The rectus femoris begins to contract concentrically just before toe-off to maximize knee extension.

*Initial swing*

After toe-off, the body is thrust into the first float phase. The line of ground reaction force at toe-off passes posterior to the knee joint, which flexes the knee as the body is propelled forward. This knee flexion is resisted by eccentric contraction of the rectus femoris, which also acts concentrically with the iliopsoas to flex the hip and advance the limb forward [11].

During initial swing, the hip abducts in relation to events that occur on the opposite side [11]. After the float phase, the opposite limb strikes the ground and the hip abductors are activated to stabilize the pelvis. As the swinging limb advances forward, pelvic rotation pushes the hip into abduction. Pelvic rotation of the swing leg also helps to place the stance leg in relative external rotation and helps initiate more supination. This motion is resisted by the hip adductors, which remain active throughout this phase.

Throughout the initial swing phase, the anterior tibialis acts concentrically to dorsiflex the ankle [11]. This action is more important in walking to clear the foot as the limb advances forward. In running, the amount of knee flexion that occurs will negate the importance of dorsiflexion to allow foot clearance.

*Terminal swing*

After the opposite limb has undergone toe-off, the second float phase occurs. At this point, the swinging limb is preparing to contact the ground. Hip flexion terminates and extension begins under concentric control of the hamstrings and gluteus maximus [11]. Knee extension occurs rapidly as a result of forward momentum and contraction of the rectus femoris. In preparation for initial contact, eccentric contraction of the hamstrings slows down knee extension at the end of terminal swing [11].

During terminal swing, the hip adducts as the foot prepares to contact the ground along the line of progression. The hip adductors concentrically bring the femur toward the midline during this portion of swing phase. They continue to be active throughout the stance phase to stabilize the lower extremity, and thereby, function throughout the entirety of the running gait cycle [23].

As the foot prepares to contact the ground, the gastrocnemius-soleus begins to contract. The anterior tibialis remains active throughout the swing phase and into a portion of the stance phase [3]. At initial contact, cocontraction of the anterior tibialis and gastrocnemius-soleus creates a stable foot for weight acceptance [11]. At this point, one complete gait cycle has occurred and the patterns that were described above are repeated as the next cycle begins.

**Running gait analysis**

As with walking gait, running gait analysis is done along a continuum from real time observational gait analysis to the use of high-resolution cameras and video recording devices; force plates; computer systems; and other laboratory measuring devices. Five gait measurement systems have been described, including motion analysis, dynamic electromyography, force plate recordings, energy cost measurements or energetics, and measurement of stride characteristics [32]. Kinetic analysis relates to force production, whereas kinematics is the measure of movement itself and reflects the effect of the kinetics [33]. Gait kinematic analysis is done best in a steady state outside of starting and stopping and requires enough space for the subject to start, walk/run, and stop [34]. Use of a treadmill allows for continuous observation and monitoring but may cause variation in movement pattern compared with nontreadmill running. Treadmill running forces runners to use a more secure gait, including spending increased time in stance phase. A recent review demonstrated that ground reaction forces, as measured by pressure-sensitive insoles in the shoes of female long-distance runners who were tested on a treadmill, were reproducible across different running velocities and stride frequencies [35]. EMG analyses across these differing running techniques varied depending on the muscle that was tested.

## Observational gait analysis

Observational gait analysis is used to some extent by all health care professionals. It is the easiest and least expensive method of analysis. Several manuals have been developed to organize and guide observational gait analysis, such as Temple University's *A Guide to a Visual Examination of Pathological Gait* or Rancho Los Amigos Medical Center's *Observational Gait Analysis Handbook* [36,37]. The gait cycle is observed with gross focus sequentially on stance, swing, and float phase. The observations are separated into subphases of stance and swing, including initial contact, loading response, midstance, and terminal stance for the stance phase, and preswing, initial swing, midswing, and terminal swing for the swing phase. Observations are made and recorded from the frontal, sagittal, and transverse views. Reflective gait markers enhance the clinician's ability to detect transverse plane abnormalities, particularly at the knee and ankle.

After the gross inspection, analysis follows an anatomic sequence, from foot and ankle to trunk, in the frontal, transverse, and sagittal planes. The observer determines deviations from normal at each joint/anatomic region and each phase/subphase. Observations of spine rotation, arm swing, and head and neck positioning also are noted.

The observational findings are summated into two areas: (1) total limb function, as described by gait deviations at each joint/phase; and (2) functional deterrents of effective weight acceptance or limb advancement [32]. The ability to pronate or weight acceptance is evaluated starting at the foot and ankle and progresses more cephalad to observe obligate motions that occur proximally—the "bottom up" approach. The ability to supinate or limb advancement is observed using a "top down" approach, and looks for proximal muscle contraction during the propulsion phases.

Excessive pronation is the most common problem that is observed on empiric running analysis. Although a physiologic amount of pronation is required, hyperpronation causes increased ground reaction forces in the medial aspect of the lower limb kinetic chain, such as the medial tibia. Muscles may need to work harder to control the excessive pronation, which may lead to tendonitis. With excessive pronation also comes excessive internal rotation of the tibia and femur. This often leads to patellofemoral maltracking. Observed excessive supination is more uncommon and can lead to increased forces on the lateral aspect of the kinetic chain. Pelvic abnormalities, such as excessive anterior and lateral tilt, also are observed frequently in runners.

## Motion analysis

In general, motion analysis provides for quantitative description of body segments in gait without quantification of forces. The simplest form of motion analysis is the use of camera for still photography or a video recording device for filming rapid events like running. Markers that are placed on the body segments allow for a more comprehensive analysis when they are imaged sequentially through a calibrated field of view. Initially, goniometers or electronically instrumented hinges were used to track limb motion [38]. Because of the changing center of knee joint motion, biaxial and triaxial systems were developed and are supplemented by a recorder that can provide immediate data on minimal and maximal arcs of motion and rates of change. More sophisticated systems have been developed in which three-dimensional coordinates can be computed by way of mathematical triangulation when two or more cameras/detectors detect the same marker. These systems are feasible to use clinically and are functionally accurate [39]. Infrared transmitters (active markers) and retro-reflective markers (passive markers) can be used without long power cords; this makes the analysis less cumbersome to set up and use. Once the computer program has calculated the motion of the limb segment, measures, such as joint angle and velocity, are calculated. Motion analysis measures can be combined with force measures to allow for calculations of joint moments, powers, and mechanical energy. There are pitfalls in patient instrumentation, marker placement, and data processing that are beyond the scope of this text that must be considered with motion analysis systems [40].

## Force plate analysis

Ground reaction forces are generated in the vertical, horizontal, and rotatory plane in conjunction with weight acceptance during stance phase. These forces—equal in intensity but opposite in direction to the forces experienced by the weight-bearing limb—can be measured with a force plate. When the measured forces are combined with information on the joint center location, ground reaction joint torques or moments can be calculated. Typically, the plate is mounted in the floor in an inconspicuous manner to avoid targeting for direct landing, which can alter desirable natural gait mechanics. Vertical loads, horizontal shear, vector patterns, joint torques, and center of pressure determinations are the most useful data from force plate analyses. Vector analysis includes sagittal plane vectors and frontal plane vectors. Gait velocity, or rate of limb loading, determines peak load [41]. Peak vertical loads of 2.5 times body weight have been measured during running [42]. Variation in running style (eg, heel-toe or foot-flat styles) impact the shape of the ground reaction force patterns [21].

### Dynamic electromyography

Muscle activity timing and relative intensity are measured with surface or fine wire needle electrodes with dynamic EMG of multiple muscles during active running or walking. Thus, dynamic EMG can be used to assess neuromuscular control of a runner. Transmission of the myoelectric signal is done by way of cable or telemetry to allow for recording. Although timing of muscle activation would seem to be a straightforward calculation, a minimum significance level for signal activation must be defined so one can decide on the onset and cessation of active contraction accurately. This minimum level has been defined as 5% of the maximal effort that is registered on manual muscle test of the muscle [43]. Cross talk from other nearby muscles can limit the accuracy of single-muscle EMG quantification, especially with surface electrodes. Computer analyses quantify muscle activity [32]. Ultimately, integration, which consists of summing the digitized, rectified signals over time, is done over short periods that are consistent with the subphases of the gait cycle.

### Energetic measurements of gait

Energy expenditure in gait is related to the alternating slowing and accelerating of body mass in conjunction with the raising and lowering center of gravity [10]. Global information on energy expenditure in normal and pathologic gait can be derived from measurements of metabolic energy expenditure and has been used to assess various pathologic gait patterns that are related to neuromuscular diseases and orthotic and prosthetic use [44]. Mechanical power has been used as a global descriptor of muscular effort, which is believed to be good surrogate of energy expenditure for gait [45]; however, several researchers have concluded that muscular effort showed no relationship with metabolic demand. Eccentric contraction is important to control the gravitational forces in a smooth, coordinated, and energy-efficient manner, primarily during stance phase. The swing phase energy expenditure may be higher than anticipated in runners [46]. The exact distribution of energy use among various muscles during human running is not known but may shed some light on running efficiency. There is no formula for the most economical running form; however, the literature on biomechanics of running gait suggests that biomechanical factors, including anthropometric dimensions, gait pattern, kinematics, and kinetics, may be related to running economy [30].

## Stride analysis

Measures of gait characteristics like cadence, speed, step length, and stride length can be useful clinically. They can be measured simply with a stopwatch or in more complex ways with apparatus like an instrumented walkway. Portable units, including insole foot switches, allow for more convenient, less expensive measures of gait characteristics. These quantitative measures, in conjunction with observational, qualitative measures, can provide a quick and easy assessment that can be repeated while tracking recovery or rehabilitation.

## Summary

Physical activity, including running, is important to general health by way of prevention of chronic illnesses and their precursors. To keep runners healthy, it is paramount that one has sound knowledge of the biomechanics of running and assessment of running gait. More so, improving performance in competitive runners is based in sound training and rehabilitation practices that are rooted firmly in biomechanical principles. This article summarized the biomechanics of running and the means with which one can evaluate running gait. The gait assessment techniques for collecting and analyzing kinetic and kinematic data can provide insights into injury prevention and treatment and performance enhancement.

## References

[1] Inman VT. The joints of the ankle. Baltimore (MD): Williams & Wilkins; 1981.
[2] Sammarco J. Biomechanics of the foot. In: Frankel VH, editor. Basic biomechanics of skeletal systems. Philadelphia: Lea & Febiger; 1980. p. 193–220.
[3] Mann RA, Baxter DE, Lutter LD. Running symposium. Foot Ankle 1981;1:190–224.
[4] Oatis CA. Biomechanics of the foot and ankle under static conditions. Phys Ther 1988;68: 1815–21.
[5] Chan CW, Rudins A. Foot biomechanics during walking and running. Mayo Clin Proc 1994; 69:448–61.
[6] Mulligan EP. Leg, ankle, and foot rehabilitation. In: Andrews JR, Harrelson GL, Wilk KE, editors. Physical rehabilitation of the injured athlete. 3rd edition. Philadelphia: WB Saunders; 2004. p. 329–76.

[7] Elftmann H. The transverse tarsal joint and its control. Clin Orthop Relat Res 1960;16:41–5.
[8] Czerniecki JM. Foot and ankle biomechanics in walking and running. Am J Phys Med Rehab 1988;67(6):246–52.
[9] Geiringer SR. Biomechanics of the running foot and related injuries. Phys Med Rehabil State Art Rev 1997;11(3):569–82.
[10] Mann RA. Biomechanics of running. In: Mack RP, editor. American Academy of Orthopaedic Surgeons Symposium on the Foot and Leg in Running Sports. St. Louis (MO): C.V. Mosby; 1982. p. 1–29.
[11] Ounpuu S. The biomechanics of walking and running. Clin Sport Med 1994;13(4):843–63.
[12] Williams KR. Biomechanics of running. Exerc Sport Sci Rev 1985;13:389–441.
[13] Putnam CA, Kozey JW. Substantive issues in running. In: Vaughan CL, editor. Biomechanics of sport. Boca Raton (FL): CRC Press; 1989. p. 1–33.
[14] Anderson T. Biomechanics and running economy. Sports Med 1996;22(2):76–89.
[15] Bates BT, Osternig LR, Mason B. Lower extremity function during the support phase of running. In: Asmussen E, Jorgensen K, editors. Biomechanics VI. Baltimore (MD): University Park Press; 1978. p. 31–9.
[16] Cavanagh PR. The shoe-ground interface in running. In: Mack PR, editor. American Academy of Orthopaedic Surgeons Symposium on the Foot and Leg in Running Sports. St. Louis (MO): Mosby; 1982. p. 30–44.
[17] Stauffer RN, Chao EY, Brewster RC. Force and motion analysis of the normal, diseased, and prosthetic ankle joint. Clin Orthop Relat Res 1977;127:189–96.
[18] Mann RA, Inman VT. Phasic activity of intrinsic muscles of the foot. J Bone Joint Surg 1964; 46A:469–81.
[19] Mann RA, Moran GT, Dougherty SE. Comparative electromyography of the lower extremity in jogging, running, and sprinting. Am J Sports Med 1986;14:501–10.
[20] Cavanagh PR. Forces and pressures between the foot and floor during normal walking and running. In: Cooper JM, Haven B, editors. Proceedings of the Biomechanics Symposium. Indianapolis (IN): Indiana University; 1980. p. 172–90.
[21] Cavanagh PR, Lafortune MA. Ground reaction forces in distance running. J Biomech 1980; 13:397–406.
[22] Dickinson JA, Cook SD, Leinhardt TM. The measurement of shock waves following heel strike while running. J Biomech 1985;18:415–22.
[23] Rodgers MM. Dynamic biomechanics of the normal foot and ankle during walking and running. Phys Ther 1988;68(12):1822–30.
[24] Adelaar RS. The practical biomechanics of running. Am J Sports Med 1986;14(6):497–500.
[25] Mann RA. Biomechanics of running. In: American Academy of Orthopaedic Surgeons Symposium on the Foot and Leg in Running Sports. St. Louis (MO): CV Mosby; 1982. p. 30–44.
[26] Winter DA. Energy generation and absorption at the ankle and knee during fast, natural, and slow cadences. Clin Orthop Relat Res 1983;175:147–54.
[27] Winter DA. Moments of force and mechanical power in jogging. J Biomech 1983;16:91–7.
[28] Morris JM. Biomechanics of the foot and ankle. Clin Orthop Relat Res 1977;122:10–7.
[29] Burdett RG. Forces predicted at the ankle during running. Med Sci Sports Exerc 1982;14: 308–16.
[30] Perry J. Anatomy and biomechanics of the hindfoot. Clin Orthop Relat Res 1983;177:9–15.
[31] Inman VT, Ralston HJ, Todd F. Human walking. Baltimore (MD): Williams & Wilkins; 1981.
[32] Perry J. Gait analysis systems. In: Gait analysis: normal and pathological function. New York: McGraw Hill; 1992. p. 349–489.
[33] Esquenazi A. Clinical application of joint kinetic analysis in gait. Phys Med Rehabil State Art Rev 2002;16(2):201–13.
[34] D'Amico E. Gait analysis systems. Phys Med Rehabil State Art Rev 2002;16(2):231–47.

[35] Karaminidis K, Arampatzis A, Bruggemann GP. Reproducibility of electromyography and ground reaction forces during various running techniques. Gait Posture 2004;19(2):115–23.

[36] Bampton S. A guide to a visual examination of pathological gait. Temple University Rehabilitation Research and Training Center #8. 1979. (Research and Training Grant #16-T-56804/3–14, Rehabilitation Services Administration Office of Human Development Services, Department of Health, Education and Welfare, Washington, DC).

[37] Pathokinesiology Department. Physical Therapy Department: Observational gait analysis handbook. Downey (CA): Professional staff association of Rancho Los Amigos Medical Center; 1989.

[38] Finley FR, Karpovich PV. Electrogoniometric analysis of normal and pathological gait. Res Quart (Suppl) 1964;5:379–84.

[39] Frigo C, Rabuffetti M, Kerrigan DC, et al. Functionally oriented and clinically feasible quantitative gait analysis method. Med Biol Eng Comput 1998;36(2):179–85.

[40] Della Croce U, Cappozzo A, Kerrigan DC. Pelvic and lower limb anatomical landmark calibration precision and its propagation to bone geometry and joint angles. Med Biol Eng Comput 1999;37(2):155–61.

[41] Skinner SR, Barnes LA, Perry J, Parker J. The relationship of gait velocity to the rate of lower extremity loading and unloading. Trans Orthop Res Soc 1980;5:273.

[42] Mann RA, Hagy J. Biomechanics of walking, running and sprinting. Am J Sports Med 1980; 8(5):345–50.

[43] Beasley WC. Quantitative muscle testing: principles and applications to research and clinical services. Arch Phys Med Rehabil 1961;42:398–425.

[44] Waters RL, Hislop HJ, Perry J, et al. Energetics: application to the study and management of locomotor disabilities. Orthop Clin N Am 1978;9:351–77.

[45] Martin PE, Morgan DW. Biomechanical considerations for economical walking and running. Med Sci Sports Exerc 1992;24(4):467–74.

[46] Marsh RL, Ellerby DJ, Carr JA, et al. Partitioning the energetics of walking and running: swinging the limbs is expensive. Science 2004;303(5654):80–3.

ELSEVIER
SAUNDERS

Phys Med Rehabil Clin N Am
16 (2005) 623–649

PHYSICAL MEDICINE
AND REHABILITATION
CLINICS OF
NORTH AMERICA

# Comprehensive Functional Evaluation of the Injured Runner

Christopher T. Plastaras, MD[a,b,*],
Joshua D. Rittenberg, MD[a,b],
Kathryn E. Rittenberg, DPT[a],
Joel Press, MD[a,b], Venu Akuthota, MD[c]

[a]Rehabilitation Institute of Chicago, Spine and Sports Rehabilitation Center,
1030 North Clark Street, Suite 500 Chicago, IL 60610, USA
[b]Northwestern University Feinberg School of Medicine,
303 East Chicago Avenue, Chicago, IL 60611, USA
[c]Department of Physical Medicine and Rehabilitation, University of Colorado
School of Medicine, P.O. Box 6510, MS F712, Aurora, CO 80045, USA

Running has been a matter of human function for many centuries; recent anthropologic research supports the fact that the bone and muscle structure of humans makes us the ideal species for endurance running [1]. This article describe the evaluation of this unique bone and muscle architecture in a functional setting. A complete evaluation that identifies the actual tissue injury and the biomechanical factors that lead to development of the injury is emphasized. A suggested sequencing of the evaluation is offered in Box 1.

## History

Often, a short office form is helpful to collect pertinent clinical information from the patient (Fig. 1). This should include a standard medical history. Additionally, specific questions about previous injuries, potential risk factors, training patterns, and goals should be asked. The athlete should be asked specifically about history of musculoskeletal injuries, such as stress fractures, tendonitis, sprains, and surgeries. For example, patients who underwent anterior cruciate ligament reconstruction with a patellar tendon donor graft may be at particular risk for patellofemoral pain [2]. Often, previous injuries can predict future injuries. A classic example is the female

* Corresponding author.
*E-mail address:* cplastaras@ric.org (C.T. Plastaras).

---

**Box 1. Sequence of the runner's evaluation**

History
Screening gait evaluation
Standing examination
   Excursion (active range of motion) tests in standing
   Strength and balance tests in standing
      Single-legged squat
      Single leg balance reach tests
      Core stability assessment
   Provocation and palliative tests in standing
      Provocation tests
      Palliative tests
Sitting examination
   Inspection and palpation
   Passive range of motion of the foot and ankle
   Knee examination
Supine examination
   Inspection and palpation
   Hip examination
   Knee examination
   Core stability assessment
Side-lying examination
Prone examination
   Subtalar neutral testing
Shoe assessment
Running assessment

---

runner who had previous stress fractures and osteopenia who is at great risk for developing new stress fractures. Runners require additional attention to issues surrounding eating habits, nutrition, and potential eating disorders. A high index of suspicion should be maintained for female athletes who have a history of eating disorders, amenorrhea, and osteoporosis—well-described as "the female triad." Risk factors for osteopenia or osteoporosis should also be collected, such as previous steroid use, caffeine intake, calcium intake, menstrual history, and family history.

History taking of the injured runner is an art form and often requires open and nonthreatening questions with knowledge of the runner's vernacular. The usual questions regarding location, duration, onset, course, exacerbating and ameliorating factors, quality, intensity, and previous treatments should be reviewed. Pain and injury can be graded based on the level of discomfort with walking, running, or rest. For example, a runner who has a tibial stress fracture usually complains of pain with running and walking [3]. If the fracture is severe, pain also may occur with rest.

## RUNNER'S EVALUATION FORM

### Training History

*Level of Competition:*
  ☐ Recreational only
  ☐ Recreational competitive
  ☐ Competitive (HS/college)
  ☐ Elite

*Years of running:* _____
*Running Club:* _____
*Pace/mile:* _____
*Mileage/week:* _____
*Long run:* _____
*Runs/week:* _____
*Shoe type:* _____
*Miles on shoe:* _____

*Running Surface:*
  ☐ Treadmill
  ☐ Street (asphalt)
  ☐ Sidewalk (concrete)
  ☐ Trail
  ☐ Track

*Cross-Training:*
  ☐ Biking
  ☐ Swimming
  ☐ Weights
  ☐ Stairs
  ☐ Yoga/Stretching
  ☐ Other:

*Shoe Insert or Orthotics:*   ☐ Yes  ☐ No
*Are you in training?:*   ☐ Yes  ☐ No    *Race and Date:* _____

*Recent change in your training?*
  ☐ Increased mileage
  ☐ New shoes or inserts
  ☐ Speed work or track work
  ☐ Hill training
  ☐ Change in terrain

*When you run, when do symptoms occur?*
  ☐ Every step of the run
  ☐ Worse toward the end of the run
  ☐ Worse at start & then improves
  ☐ Only after the run ends (next day)

### Medical History

*Date and Description of Injury:* _____
*Previous Treatments for Injury:* _____
*Past Medical & Surgical History:* _____
*Medications:* _____
*Allergies:* _____
*Prior Musculoskeletal Injuries:* _____

*History of stress fractures:*   ☐ Yes  ☐ No
　　　　　　　steroid use:   ☐ Yes  ☐ No
　　　　　　　osteoporosis:   ☐ Yes  ☐ No
　　　　　　　eating disorders:   ☐ Yes  ☐ No

*Female History:*   ☐ N/A
　reg. periods:   ☐ Yes  ☐ No
　pregnant:   ☐ Yes  ☐ No
　age of 1st period: _____
　date of last period: _____

Fig. 1. Runner's evaluation intake sheet.

Conversely, pain that improves after warm up but worsens following a run may be more consistent with a tendinopathy.

Training errors are the most common source of running injuries [4]. Injured runners often attempt to train "too much, too soon, too fast." Therefore, the athlete's training habits should be investigated in detail. An increasing injury rate has been correlated directly to increased mileage per week, particularly if the athlete runs more than 20 miles per week [5]. A sudden and rapid increase of running mileage is a frequent training error.

In our experience, college freshmen runners are a high-risk group for injuries; their bodies are not conditioned for an often sudden, and rapid, increase to the 70 to 100 miles per week training program that is popular with elite training regimens. Athletes who participate in "speed work" also are at risk for developing overuse injuries. These shorter duration, increased intensity workouts—which frequently incorporate track sprints—require physical demands on the musculoskeletal system that many endurance athletes are not yet ready to perform. In addition, athletes who train on a treadmill during colder winter months and then transition suddenly to land-based running in the spring frequently encounter injuries. The treadmill cushions shock and assists the contact foot to propel backward, which differentiates it from land-based running. Runners who started a hill or interval training program abruptly also may encounter musculoskeletal problems. Additionally, runners who train on cambered (slanted) surfaces or sand also may be at risk for injury. Questions about warm up, flexibility training, strength training, and cross-training should also be included in the evaluation.

## Physical examination

The physical examination of the injured runner must reach beyond the site of tissue injury. The easy part of the examination is identifying the injured structure. Often, runners will come in already knowing their diagnosis because of previous experience, running magazines, books, and web surfing. The more difficult and more important part of the evaluation is identifying the offending biomechanical factors that caused the injury. A treatment strategy can be developed based on the functional deficits that are noted. Muscle imbalances that are common to runners should be identified. In particular, tight soleus/inhibited anterior tibialis and tight hip flexor/inhibited gluteus maximus are common patterns that are seen in runners.

The clinician needs to develop a sequence or flow to the examination, usually starting with a screening gait evaluation and then transitioning to observations while the patient is standing, sitting, supine, side-lying, and prone (see Box 1). A thorough site-specific examination will be performed based on the location of pain. Typically, actual running is assessed last. In runners, routine manual muscle testing is not a sensitive measure of strength deficits. Therefore, the clinician needs to make every attempt to challenge the athlete in weight-bearing and functional positions to uncover deficits. Often, the problem is not apparent until the athlete is fatigued adequately. Runners should be undressed and exposed properly to perform a comprehensive examination. Rolling up a pant leg is unacceptable. This article describes a general framework for the clinician who is examining an injured runner.

## Screening gait evaluation

The walking gait analysis is an extremely powerful screening tool. In fact, seasoned clinicians often can make the diagnosis and pick up pertinent biomechanical factors just with careful observation of gait. The screening gait evaluation starts by asking the patient to walk at a comfortable pace without shoes or socks. Gait should be analyzed from the front, back, and lateral views. First, take note of any obvious asymmetries or antalgic gait patterns. This gives information about possible leg length discrepancy, major joint restriction, or profound muscle weakness. For example, the oft-seen Trendelenburg gait indicates gluteus medius weakness. Next, use a systematic approach to analyze each region of the body. Often, a bottom-up approach is selected, looking at the feet and then progressing proximally. Look for proper heel strike, degree and timing of subtalar and midfoot pronation in loading, as well as supination of the foot in terminal stance. Excessive or prolonged pronation causes obligate tibial and femoral internal rotation which may lead to patellofemoral pain [6]. Video analysis with freeze frame capability can act as a useful adjunct to the clinical gait analysis. Markers may be placed over landmarks, such as the tibial tuberosity, midpatella, and distal femur, to facilitate knee joint frontal plane observation [7].

During the screening gait evaluation, certain gait exaggerations may help to make deficits more easily observable [8]. Long stride gait observation is useful to assess the subject's ability for rear leg loading in late stance (Fig. 2). The subject should be able to bring his/her center of mass over the foot. This tweak is invaluable in assessing the degree of hip extension and

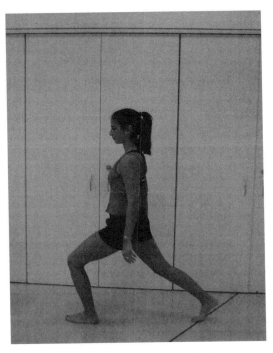

Fig. 2. Long stride exaggerated gait.

ankle dorsiflexion. A tight hip flexor causes the subject to decrease stride length, limit hip extension, and increase lumbar lordosis. Early heel rise is seen commonly when there is a lack of ankle dorsiflexion, as with gastrosoleus tightness. The exaggerated crouch gait helps to evaluate pronation (shock-absorbing ability), mainly in the sagittal plane (Fig. 3). For example, if the foot and ankle remain in a supinated position through the crouched gait, poor pronation should be suspected. Again, early heel rise occurs with gastrocnemius tightness. Additionally, an exaggerated arm swing gait can be used to assess how the trunk and pelvis are moving in proper sequence. The subject is directed to clasp his/her hands together in front of the body and swing the arms from side to side in the transverse plane while walking. The trunk and pelvis are observed for normal reciprocal movement. Abdominal muscle recruitment problems may arise if the reciprocal pattern is not occurring.

Finally, athletes are asked to walk on their toes and to walk on their heels. When walking on their toes, the plantar flexion active range of motion and strength is assessed. Observing a relative calcaneal inversion at the end range of plantar flexion indicates proper posterior tibialis muscle firing [9].

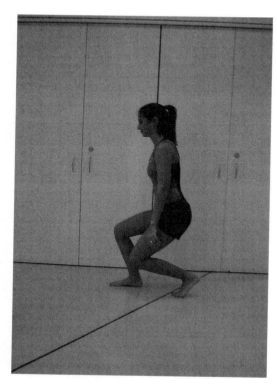

Fig. 3. Exaggerated crouch gait.

Walking on the heels evaluates ankle dorsiflexion active range of motion and strength.

## Standing examination

The primary objective of this part of the examination is to assess the alignment and posture of the spine, pelvis, and lower limb. Runners are observed standing with double leg support in all three planes. The major landmarks are the iliac crest, posterior superior iliac spine, anterior superior iliac spine greater trochanter, lateral malleolus, and the calcaneus. Excessive anterior or posterior pelvic tilt (sagittal plane) can be appreciated when viewing from the side. Frontal plane observations can detect pelvic obliquities and leg length discrepancies. The putative "miserable malalignment syndrome" can be observed in this position. Typically, this is seen in susceptible female runners as increased femoral anteversion, vastus medialis oblique (VMO) atrophy, wide Q angle, and foot pronation. Meisser et al [10] correlated a standing or functional Q-angle of greater than 16° to patellofemoral pain in runners. If desired, VMO atrophy can be measured by taking a circumferential girth of both distal quadriceps. A difference of more than 1 cm can indicate significant quadriceps atrophy [11]. In addition, leg length discrepancy may be a source of injury in runners and should be suspected if there is asymmetrical weight bearing, hip external rotation, knee flexion, and pronation in standing. Patients who have patellofemoral pain also may exhibit "grasshopper eyes" patellae (externally rotated due to patella alta) or "squinting" patellae (internally rotated).

In the static standing position, the foot and ankle can be observed for pes planus (flat foot) or pes cavus (high arched). Viewing the patient directly behind the ankles may show "too many toes" (lateral three toes are visible) which indicates excessive pronation or hip external rotation (Fig. 4). Although pes planus is more common and a relative risk factor for running

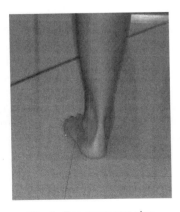

Fig. 4. Too many toes sign.

injuries, the existence of pes cavus seems to be a much higher predictor of an overuse running injury [12]. The degree of pes planus can be determined by the navicular drop test, in which the navicular location is assessed in the subtalar neutral position and then with weight bearing. A decrease of greater than 1.5 cm is considered to significant pes planus [13].

## Excursion (active range of motion) tests in standing

Active range of motion of the lower limb and spine can be assessed in standing to get a better idea of a runner's true excursion. A "bottom-up" approach is used, assessing the foot and ankle range first and then progressing to the knee and hip. First, the first metatarsophalangeal (MTP) range of motion is assessed by having the runner actively extend the big toe. Elite runners need an active range of motion of at least 45° of MTP extension to achieve a powerful push-off [14]. Second, a weight-bearing supination and pronation excursion test is done by having the runner plant heels and toes to the ground and then attempt to maximally invert and evert the calcaneus. The first ray should point straight ahead to avoid compensation through the forefoot. Any asymmetry of subtalar motion should be noted. The subtalar neutral position (see later discussion), also can be found in this weight-bearing position. Third, a double leg squat (allowing for the heels to leave the ground) is used to record the knee flexion and ankle dorsiflexion active range. Individuals who have tight soleus muscles demonstrate excessive hip flexion (to maintain their center of gravity over their foot) and an early heel rise. Double leg squat additionally screens for knee abnormalities, such as patellofemoral and meniscal pathology. Fourth, the hip crossover tests are performed to assess the range of hip internal and external rotation (Fig. 5). Finally, the lumbosacral spine motion testing is performed and recorded.

## Strength and balance tests in standing

### Single-legged squat

Single leg stance and squat test (also termed single-legged squat) is the single most useful and valid dynamic standing test [15]. In this test, runners are asked to lower themselves as far as possible and then return to a standing position without losing balance. The initial frontal plane observation is to detect weak hip abductors by way of a Trendelenburg sign (Fig. 6). Then athletes should be observed performing this maneuver in the sagittal and transverse planes. Excessive hip adduction has been noted in asymptomatic women who perform this test and may represent a risk factor for hip and knee injuries [15]. A lack of knee control also may be demonstrated with this test, termed a "knee wobble." Increased hip adduction and knee wobbling may be a sign of gluteal muscle weakness in the frontal and transverse planes.

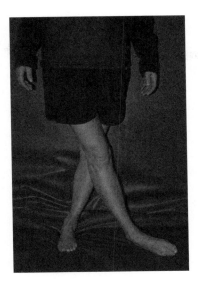

Fig. 5. Hip crossover test.

*Single leg balance reach tests*

Single leg balance reach tests incorporate a single leg squat with a reach in the sagittal, coronal, and transverse planes (Fig. 7) [16]. These tests further help the clinician to identify the planes of motion that are difficult and ones that are preferred. The patient is instructed to stand on one leg and reach the other foot in front of them as far as they are able, but without touching the ground. The same instruction is given to the side (coronal plane) and the side and back with twisting (transverse plane). Frequently, runners perform well with single leg reaches in the sagittal plane but perform much worse with reaches in the frontal and transverse planes. During these reach tests, hindfoot motion can be observed for asymmetry, which indicates restrictions of the subtalar joint or talocrural joint. Reach tests also may reveal weakness of the gluteal muscles—attested by a pelvic drop—and weakness of eccentric quadriceps, often with a compensatory forward trunk lean. Weak hip abductors correlated with iliotibial band syndrome in long distance runners [17]. Commonly, early heel rise on the stance leg can indicate a shortened, weakened soleus muscle. If the athlete is not challenged with reach tests, single leg step downs can be used (Fig. 8). The beauty of these tests is that they also can be used as effective therapeutic exercises [17].

*Core stability assessment*

The core stability assessment is started by observing the qualitative mistakes made with a power runner pose (Fig. 9). This may include a pelvic drop, knee internal rotation, or excessive foot and ankle pronation. A sophisticated standing core muscle assessment is described by Geraci and

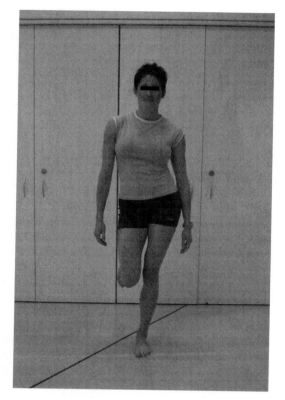

Fig. 6. Trendelenburg sign with single-legged squat.

Brown elsewhere in this volume. In essence, the core muscles are assessed in standing in all three planes.

### Provocation and palliative tests in standing

#### Provocation tests

Hopping on a single leg (hop test) can be used as a provocation test for stress fractures or other bony abnormalities, such as stress fractures. Additionally, the single and double leg squats that were performed earlier serve as a screen for knee, hip, and talocrural pathology. Walking in a deep knee crouch ("duck walking") has been used in preparticipation examinations for years as a screen for meniscal pathology. Plantar fasciitis may be detected by having the runner exaggerate propulsion at terminal stance to mimic a windlass maneuver.

#### Palliative tests

If pain is provoked during the single leg squat, relieving maneuvers can be performed to ascertain a biomechanical cause. The hip assistance

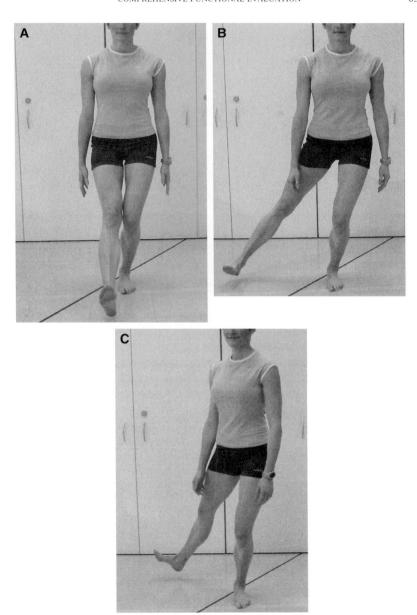

Fig. 7. Balance reach tests in sagittal (*A*), frontal (*B*), and transverse planes (*C*).

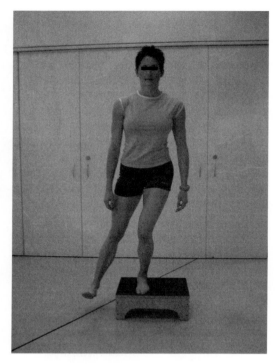

Fig. 8. Step down in the transverse plane (also known as the pelvic drop exercise).

palliative maneuver is performed by forcefully compressing the pelvic girdle by pushing the greater trochanters together as the patient performs a single leg squat (Fig. 10a). Medial patellar glide is a palliative maneuver that is performed by manually guiding the kneecap medially as the patient squats on the painful knee (Fig. 10b). This can be done more formally by applying tape [18]. Finally, a medial arch support (eg, orthosis, your cupped hand, wadded sock) also can serve as a palliative device (Fig. 10c). Pain should be monitored during each of the three maneuvers. Decrement of pain on any of these palliative tests can help to convince the clinician and the patient that intervention at that part of the kinetic chain should be addressed. For example, if pain resolves with hip assistance, functional gluteal strengthening should be a focus of rehabilitation. If medial patellar compression helps, patellar taping should be considered. If medial arch support helps, a motion control shoe or foot orthoses may be helpful.

## Seated examination

### Inspection and palpation

In addition to checking routine strength, sensation, reflexes, and seated slump tests, the seated position offers a good opportunity to do an

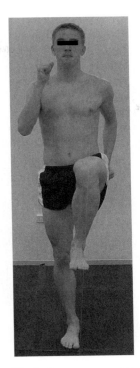

Fig. 9. Power runner pose.

unloaded foot and ankle examination. First, the runner's feet should be inspected for calluses, necrotic toe nails, and blisters. In the runner who has foot and ankle pain, a thorough palpation examination can pinpoint tissue injury (Table 1). If pain is noted around the base of the fifth metatarsal, a careful palpation examination and radiograph is required to distinguish peroneal tendonitis, avulsion fracture of the base of the fifth metatarsal, and a diaphyseal (Jones') fracture [19]. Jones' fracture often needs to be treated with pinning because of frequent nonunion. Dorsal tenderness with a Tinel's sign between the third and fourth metatarsals distally is pathognomonic for a Morton's neuroma. The Windlass maneuver, in which the first MTP and the ankle are dorsiflexed maximally, can bring out the plantar fascia [20].

*Passive range of motion of the foot and ankle*

An open kinetic chain assessment of the foot and ankle joint passive range of motion can yield areas where joint mobilization can be helpful. Subtalar joint mobility is assessed passively by placing the joint in neutral position then inverting and everting the calcaneus (Fig. 11). Careful note should be made of side to side difference. Restricted subtalar eversion is

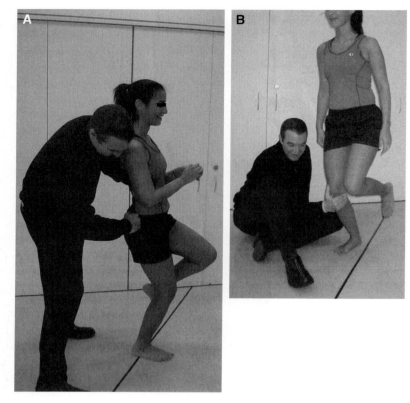

Fig. 10. Palliative tests. (*A*) Hip assistance. (*B*) Medial patellar glide. (*C*) Medial arch support.

common and may cause problems with shock absorption (pronation) during the loading response of the stance phase of running [21,22].

Talocrural joint mobility along with gastrocnemius and soleus flexibility should be assessed. Runners frequently have a tight gastrosoleus complex. Because the gastrocnemius crosses two joints, it is particularly vulnerable to developing tightness. In the authors' experience, however, the soleus is frequently just as tight as the gastrocnemius in runners. The gastrocnemius length can be measured by dorsiflexing the foot with the knee straight, and the soleus length can be measured by dorsiflexing the foot with the knee bent. Tightness in the gastrosoleus complex (ankle equinus) can lead to a compensatory midfoot and subtalar pronation [23]. Ankle equinus can lead to several running injuries, including plantar fasciitis, Achilles tendinopathy, and medial tibial stress syndrome [23,24]. It is believed that runners require at least 15° to 20° of dorsiflexion for efficient running [9].

Midtarsal motion is assessed with the calcaneus in eversion. This essentially places the midtarsal joints in parallel and unlocks the midfoot (Fig. 12). Midtarsal motion should be eliminated by placing the calcaneus in

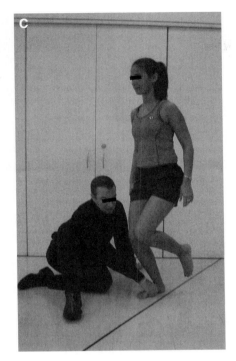

Fig. 10 (*continued*)

inversion. A flexible midfoot in calcaneal inversion and eversion may require orthotic inversion.

Finally, first ray joint play and first MTP joint passive range of motion should be assessed. The first ray joint play is assessed by determining if the

Table 1
Overuse injuries of the foot and ankle based on site of tenderness

| Site of tenderness | Diagnosis |
| --- | --- |
| Achilles tendon and paratendon | Achilles tendonitis |
| Posterior heel (calcaneus) tenderness | Calcaneal stress fracture or severe disease (in adolescent) |
| Retrocalcaneal bursa | Retrocalcaneal bursitis |
| Medial calcaneal tuberosity | Plantar fasciitis |
| Tarsal tunnel | Extrinsic flexor tendonitis |
| Anterior talofibular ligament | Lateral ankle sprain or sinus tarsi syndrome |
| Talar dome | Talus stress fracture or osteochondritis dissecans |
| Proximal dorsal aspect of navicular (N-spot) | Navicular stress fracture |
| Base of 5th metatarsal | Jones' fracture, peroneal tendonitis |
| Lateral midfoot | Cuboid syndrome |
| Shaft of metatarsals | March fracture |
| Sesamoid | Sesamoiditis or stress fracture |

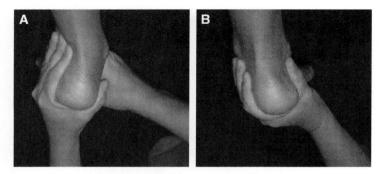

Fig. 11. Subtalar inversion (*A*) and inversion (*B*) testing with the foot unweighted.

first metatarsal is aligned with the other metatarsals (neutral) or if it is dorsiflexed or plantarflexed in relation to the other metatarsals.

*Knee examination*

In sitting, runners who have knee pain should be assessed for crepitus and patellar tracking. The runner is asked to extend the knee from 90° of flexion to full extension. The patella disengages from the trochlea at the end range of extension; however, if the patella abruptly disengages laterally, this is termed a positive "J-sign." Patella alta and a prominent Hoffa's pad should be noted because these conditions may predispose runners to patellofemoral pain. In runners who are suspected to have a femoral stress fracture, a femoral fulcrum test should be performed. With this test, one arm is used as a lever point underneath the posterior thigh and the other pushes down on the distal thigh. The seated position offers a good opportunity to palpate the patellar tendon from its origin at the inferior pole of the patella to its

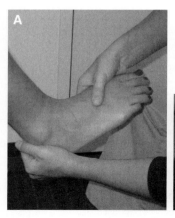
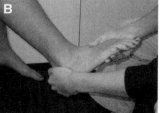

Fig. 12. Midfoot motion. (*A*) With hindfoot locked in supination (calcaneal inversion). (*B*) With hindfoot unlocked in pronation (calcaneal eversion).

attachment at the tibial tuberosity. It can be made to stand out by having the runner actively extend the knee, and then the examiner presses down on the superior pole of the patella. Adolescent athletes frequently have traction apophysitis at this location (eg, inferior pole of patella = Sinding-Larsen-Johansson syndrome; tibial tuberosity = Osgood-Schlater syndrome). Typically, the rest of the knee and thigh examination takes place in the supine position.

## Supine examination

### Inspection and palpation

In supine, pelvic landmarks and leg lengths should be reassessed. Straight leg raise is done to assess further for adverse dynamic neural tension and hamstring length. In runners who have shin splints, a palpation examination of the medial tibia can help to differentiate stress fractures from soft tissue injury. Localized, rather than diffuse, pain with palpation and percussion may be a sign of a tibial stress fracture [3].

### Hip examination

Passive range of motion testing of hip flexion, abduction, internal rotation, and external rotation is assessed in the supine position. The modified Thomas test is a valuable test that should be performed to assess the muscle length of the iliopsoas, tensor fascia lata, and rectus femoris (Fig. 13). Recreational runners frequently encounter problems with tight hip

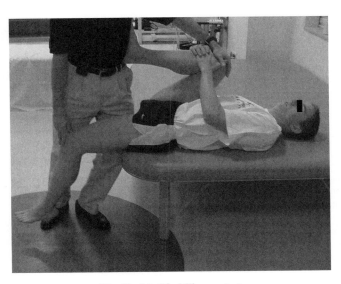

Fig. 13. Modified Thomas test.

flexors and quadriceps. A lack of hip internal rotation and abduction may warrant a work-up for hip intra-articular pathology. Provocation tests for hip intra-articular pathology include hip internal rotation with overpressure, flexion-abduction-external rotation (FABER) test, and hip scour test. There are innumerable sacroiliac joint provocation tests that can be performed in supine, side-lying, and prone. No single test has proven to be better than others [25]; however, the authors use the Patrick test, thigh thrust, and Gaenslen test frequently.

*Knee examination*

The supine examination also includes a thorough evaluation of the knee. Standard knee tests to evaluate for swelling, ligamentous laxity, and meniscal or intra-articular pathology [26] are performed. Finding and palpating the site of tenderness can help to narrow the differential diagnosis (Table 2). Clarke's test (patellar grind) should be performed to evaluate for patellofemoral pain syndrome. Crossley et al [27] described a three-dimensional method for assessing the mobility and orientation of the patella. This assessment should be done if patellar taping is a consideration. The Noble compression test is a provocative test for iliotibial band syndrome. Typically, this test is performed supine; however, it can be sensitized by performing it in single leg stance (Fig. 14). Tibial torsion can be assessed in the supine position. The knee is placed in the frontal plane by placing the femoral condyles in line, then an imaginary line is drawn between the tibial malleoli. This angle of inclination from the frontal plane becomes the amount of tibial torsion. The most common tibial alignment abnormality is bowleggedness or tibia varum.

*Core stability assessment*

In the supine position, core stability can be assessed qualitatively by performing a pelvic bridge. The pelvic bridge requires gluteal, hamstring, and

Table 2
Overuse injuries of the knee based on site of tenderness

| Site of Tenderness | Diagnosis |
| --- | --- |
| Gerdy's tubercle | Iliotibial band syndrome |
| Lateral femoral epicondyle | Iliotibial band syndrome |
| Inferior pole of patella | Patellar tendonitis, Sinding-Larsen-Johansson |
| Superior pole of patella | Quadriceps tendonitis |
| Tibial tuberosity | Osgood-Schlater |
| Medial band | Plica syndrome |
| Joint lines | Menisceal pathology |
| Patellar facets | Patellofemoral pain syndrome |
| Retinaculum | Patellofemoral pain syndrome |
| Fat pad | Hoffa's fat pain syndrome |

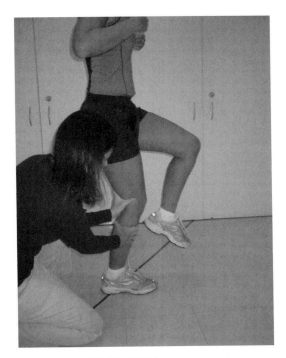

Fig. 14. Modified Noble compression test.

paraspinal strength. If a proper posterior pelvic tilt is done in addition to the pelvic bridge, abdominal muscles also will need to be engaged. Hamstring cramping during the pelvic bridge can be a subjective sign of gluteal underuse and hamstring overuse. During the bridge, the runner can be asked to extend one leg, balancing on just one planted leg. A side to side difference can be indicative of hip girdle muscle weakness. The upper abdominals of the core can be assessed by having the athlete go from a supine position to a long sit position. Compensatory maneuvers include leading with neck flexion and lifting of the heels. The lower abdominals can be tested using the leg lowering test that was described by Kendall et al [28]. The athlete is asked to keep a reduced lumbar lordosis as he/she lowers the legs from 90° of hip flexion. The hip flexion range in which the athlete returns to lumbar lordosis is recorded. Athletes who have adequate lower abdominal strength should be able to maintain their back flat for at least 45° of hip flexion. These tests serve as an augment to the standing core stability assessment.

## Side-lying examination

In this position, the greater trochanter is palpated easily for tenderness or swelling. Manual muscle testing of the hip external rotators and abductors can be performed in the side-lying position. Failure to detect any weakness on manual muscle testing is common in this unloaded position, however, and findings should be compared with the evaluation in the standing position. During resisted hip abduction, the subject frequently will "cheat" by using hip flexor muscles to provide more power. An easy way of sensitizing this test is to perform it with the subject abducting with the hip internally rotated—using more the tensor fascia lata—versus externally rotated—using more of the gluteus medius. More commonly, weakness is seen only when the subject is tested in an externally rotated position. The modified Ober test also is performed to evaluate for iliotibial band tightness (Fig. 15) [28].

**Prone examination**

Posterior to anterior glide along the lumbar spine and pelvis may indicate discogenic pain, sacroiliac joint–mediated pain, and sacral stress injury. The prone position is an opportunity to perform Ely test for rectus femoris tightness, a common finding in runners. Femoral stretch testing should be performed by passively bending the individual's knee then adding hip extension as a sensitizing maneuver. Like any dural tension test, the femoral stretch is considered positive if concordant symptoms are reproduced, worsens with dural tension tautness, and improves with dural tension slackening. A formal assessment of femoral torsion (femoral anteversion) can be done in the prone position, particularly if a miserable malalignment syndrome is seen in standing. The knee is flexed to 90° and then the examiner internally rotates the hip until the greater trochanter becomes palpably prominent. The angle of the tibia from vertical becomes the amount of femoral anteversion [29]. Radiographs often are needed to confirm femoral anteversion. Increased femoral internal (medial) torsion causes in-toeing [26].

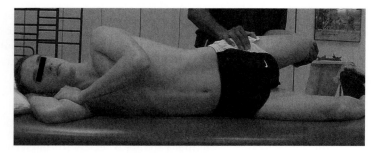

Fig. 15. Modified Ober test.

*Subtalar neutral testing*

The prone position offers the ideal opportunity to assess for the so-called "subtalar neutral position." The subtalar neutral position is found by placing the thumb and index finger on the anterior talus, and then moving the calcaneus until talonavicular congruency (talus is felt equally by both fingers) is found (Fig. 16). The importance of the finding of the subtalar neutral position has diminished for multiple reasons. First, the neutral typically is looked for in the open kinetic chain position, which is not a functional position for runners. Second, the assumption that the subtalar neutral is the most efficient and effective position for running has not been validated. The authors use subtalar neutral testing to identify the relationships of the hindfoot to the forefoot and the lower leg. In the authors' experience, runners who have certain foot types need custom foot orthoses more frequently.

## Shoe assessment

Running shoes have evolved into high-tech equipment that often obviates the need for foot orthoses; however, ill-fitting or worn-out running shoes can contribute to overuse injuries [30]. A comprehensive evaluation of the runner involves looking at the athlete's current and previous pairs of shoes; therefore, the authors ask that runners bring their last two pairs of shoes to the initial evaluation (Box 2).

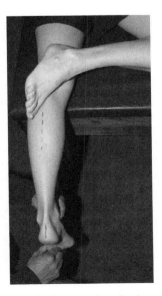

Fig. 16. Subtalar neutral testing in prone.

---

**Box 2. Shoe assessment**

Determine age and mileage of shoe
Determine if shoe is too tight or too loose for the size of the foot
Look at last: straight versus curved
Look at shoe torsion: stiffness
Look for anti-pronation materials: foot bridge or medial arch
   materials
Look at heel counter and height
Look for shock-absorbing material
Look at lacing technique
Determine type of shoe
Determine wear patterns: asymmetry
Determine if type of shoe matches foot type

---

Running shoes can be divided into three general types: (1) motion control (antipronation), (2) stability (neutral), and (3) shock absorbing (cushioning). The most important determination to make is if the examinee's foot type fits his/her current pair of running shoes. The age and mileage on the shoes should be ascertained. In general, running shoes tend to wear down after 300 to 500 miles. Shock-absorbing shoes tend to wear down more quickly than motion control shoes, especially if running on wet surfaces and if they are more than 1 year old. Often, runners get shoes that are tight because they fit their shoes with considering the swelling of the foot with running. Shoes that are too loose also can cause problems, such as pistoning of the heel out of the shoe. Certain lacing techniques can help to prevent pistoning and alleviate pressure from the dorsum of the foot.

The last of the shoe also should be determined. The last refers to the material between the shoe and sole as well as the stitching on the material. Individuals who have hyperpronation require a straight-stitched board last, whereas runners who have high-arched feet require a curved-stitched slip last. The amount of midfoot motion that is available with the shoe can be determined by twisting the shoe along its transverse crease. Hyperpronating runners require a stiffer shoe. A stiffer shoe often has antipronation materials, such as so-called "foot bridges" and hard medial arch materials. The heel counter design also can help to control the hindfoot in runners who have heel contact on initial contact (slower runners). Faster runners should not have a heel counter that is built up excessively.

The wear patterns on an older shoe also can offer clues in determining if the shoe fits the foot type. Normally, hindfoot (initial contact) runners have some wear at the lateral portion of the heel because stance phase begins with a supinated foot position. After initial contact, the foot pronates before supinating again. If excessive wear is seen on the lateral aspect of the forefoot, a pes cavus foot with inability to pronate should be suspected. Asymmetric pronation also can be suspected if the heel and midfoot has more medial wear than the other shoe. The most common mistakes that the authors see is that runners get shoes that prevent physiologic pronation and shock absorption. Finally, the lacing technique that is used can help to make the shoe fit the foot more adequately.

**Running analysis**

Running gait analysis should be a routine evaluation tool for the treating team. When assessing running, it is important to remember that running is biomechanically different than walking and that treadmill running is different than road running. Compared with walking, running requires a greater joint range of motion and has greater eccentric muscle demand. Initial heel contact position varies, depending on speed; slower runners land on their heels, whereas sprinters land on their forefoot. Often in the clinic setting, a treadmill is a convenient way to watch athletes run; however, a video of the runner viewed in multiple planes provides the truest picture of the running form. In the authors' experience, reflective gait markers further enhance the clinician's ability to detect transverse plane abnormalities, particularly at the knee and ankle.

A systematic running analysis that evaluates each joint in all three planes is suggested. Initially, observe the runner's arm swing and posture. Take note of arm position, direction, and amount of swing. Asymmetric or abnormal arm swing may be the result or the cause of a distal kinetic chain dysfunction. Posturally, runners may have an increased lumbar lordosis when compared with walking gait. This often is an indicator of tight hip flexors or inefficient use of abdominal muscles. Stride length should be observed for the amount of hip extension. A forward trunk lean (anterior pelvic tilt) also may be a compensation for tight hip flexors or weak gluteal muscles. Anterior pelvic tilting causes an increased knee flexion angle, and thus, produces more eccentric force loads on the quadriceps [23]. Abnormal pelvic dynamics also may be evident with a lateral pelvic tilt (Trendelenburg sign) during running.

The quality of knee control is determined in the sagittal, frontal, and transverse planes. In the sagittal plane, excessive knee flexion may occur with hamstring tightness or excessive anterior pelvic tilt. In the frontal plane, genu valgus (knee abduction) can be seen. In the transverse plane, control of the obligate tibial and femoral internal rotation with pronation should be observed.

Particular attention is paid to the foot and ankle. Runners are assessed for normal pronation, hyperpronation, or inadequate pronation. In the frontal plane, the calcaneus is observed for adequate and symmetric eversion after initial contact. Adequate pronation allows for attenuation of forces at the foot in loading. Lack of subtalar eversion often prevents

Table 3
Running injuries synopsis

| | Greater trochanteric pain | Patellofemoral pain syndrome | Iliotibial band syndrome | Tibial stress fracture | Medial tibial stress syndrome | Plantar fasciitis |
|---|---|---|---|---|---|---|
| Pathognomonic physical examination findings | Tender greater trochanter<br><br>Weak gluteus medius | Positive Clark's sign; relief of symptoms with hip assist, medial patellar compression, or arch assist (see figures)<br><br>Weak gluteus medius; tight gastroc-soleus, hip flexors | Noble's compression, Ober's test<br><br>Weak gluteus medius | Pain with single leg hop, focal tenderness on tibia<br><br>May have dynamic hyper-pronation of midfoot | Diffuse tenderness medial to tibial crest<br><br>Dynamic hyper-pronation of midfoot | Tender inferior medial calcaneus |
| Clinical symptom complex | Pain in lateral hip pain | Anterior knee pain especially going downstairs, Theatre sign | Lateral knee pain, especially worse toward end of run | Complaints of "shin splints" every step of run | Complaints of "shin splints" improve during run | Medial heel pain, especially first step in the morning |
| Tissue injury complex | Gluteus medius or tensor fascia lata tendonitis | Patellar cartilage (chondromalacia) and synovium | ITB tendinopathy or possible bursitis at lateral femoral condyle | Tibial cortical bone | Tibial periosteum at muscle origin of soleus/posterior tibialis | Plantar fascia inflammation |
| Functional biomechanical deficits | Weak gluteus medius; tight TFL/iliopsoas | Tight ITB, rectus femoris, iliopsoas, gastroc-soleus; weakness of gluteus medius, rigid subtalar eversion | Tight ITB, rectus femoris, iliopsoas, gastroc-soleus; weakness of gluteus medius, rigid subtalar eversion | Tight and weak soleus | Tight and weak soleus | Tight and weak soleus; hallux rigidus |
| Functional adaptation complex | Compensated Trendelenburg gait, sometimes pelvic obliquity | Incongruence of femoral and tibial internal rotation loading response (causing lateral patellar tracking) | Compensated Trendelenburg gait, sometimes pelvic obliquity | Rigid subtalar eversion; dynamic hyperpronation of midfoot | Rigid subtalar eversion; dynamic hyper-pronation of midfoot | Rigid subtalar eversion; tight hip flexors |

| | Tensor fascia lata and iliotibial band | Tensor fascia lata and iliotibial band; lateral retinaculum stress | Tensor fascia lata and iliotibial band | Posterior tibialis muscle origination | Posterior tibialis muscle origination | Posterior tibialis |
|---|---|---|---|---|---|---|
| Tissue overload complex | Tensor fascia lata and iliotibial band | Tensor fascia lata and iliotibial band; lateral retinaculum stress | Tensor fascia lata and iliotibial band | Posterior tibialis muscle origination | Posterior tibialis muscle origination | Posterior tibialis |
| Gait findings | Compensated Trendelenburg, external rotation of foot | Hyperpronation | Compensated Trendelenburg | Antalgic gait | External rotation of foot | Early heel rise |
| Radiograph | Normal | Normal; sunrise views may show patella positioned laterally in femoral groove | Normal | May have cortical thickening after 2 weeks | Normal | Normal or calcaneal spur |
| MRI | Gluteus medius tendinosis or greater trochanter bursa formation | Normal or early patellar cartilaginous changes | Normal or increased signal at distal ITB near lateral femoral condyle | Increased signal intensity on STIR images [31] | Diffuse signal intensity of tibial periosteum | Normal or increased signal on T2-images of plantar fascia |
| Ultrasound | Gluteus medius tendinosis or greater trochanter bursa formation | Normal | Normal or thickened ITB, hypoechoic at distal ITB near lateral femoral condyle | May be painful at site of fracture | Negative | Negative or thickening |
| Bone scan | Negative | Negative | Negative | Focal increased uptake | Fusiform increased uptake | Diffuse, nonspecific increased uptake |
| Rehab pearls | Closed chain gluteal muscle strength and dynamic balance | Patellar taping early; closed chain gluteal muscle strength and dynamic balance | Gluteus medius strengthening, Functional triplanar stretching [17] | Consider pool running or harness-supported running to maintain cardiovascular fitness | "Stomp the bug"; subtalar mobilization; motion control shoe | "Stomp the bug"; subtalar mobilization; frozen golf balls |

ITB, iliotibial band; STIR, short T1 inversion recovery.

adequate shock absorption and places excessive strain on kinetically linked structures, such as the knee or hip. Greater vertical impact forces and delayed pronation have been implicated as risk factors for running-related injuries [21,31]. Often, a medial heel whip (during swing phase) running style is seen in runners who have prolonged foot pronation. A lateral heel whip, seen less commonly, results from excessive supination.

## Summary

In most cases, a detailed history provides the information that is necessary for the clinician to diagnose the injured runner correctly; however, to treat the injury and guide a successful rehabilitation program, the physical examination must go beyond the standard regional musculoskeletal examination. The victims (tissue injury) and the culprits (biomechanical deficits) must be identified to facilitate treatment (Table 3). Gait and other dynamic assessments help to reveal underlying deficits in function that may have contributed to injury. In short, the entire functional kinetic chain must be considered and weak links identified.

## References

[1] Bramble DM, Lieberman DE. Endurance running and the evolution of *Homo*. Nature 2004; 432(7015):345–52.
[2] Eriksson K, Anderberg P, Hamberg P, et al. There are differences in early morbidity after ACL reconstruction when comparing patellar tendon and semitendinosus tendon graft. A prospective randomized study of 107 patients. Scand J Med Sci Sports 2001;11(3):170–7.
[3] Fredericson M, Bergman AG, Hoffman KL, et al. Tibial stress reaction in runners. Correlation of clinical symptoms and scintigraphy with a new magnetic resonance imaging grading system. Am J Sports Med 1995;23(4):472–81.
[4] James SL, Bates BT, Osternig LR. Injuries to runners. Am J Sports Med 1978;6(2):40–50.
[5] Macera CA. Lower extremity injuries in runners. Advances in prediction. Sports Med 1992; 13(1):50–7.
[6] Powers CM. The influence of altered lower-extremity kinematics on patellofemoral joint dysfunction: a theoretical perspective. J Orthop Sports Phys Ther 2003;33(11):639–46.
[7] O'Connor A, Zemon D. Observational gait analysis tool. Presented at Sports Rehabilitation Medicine XV Chicago, April 2004.
[8] Gray G. Chain reaction festival. Adrian (MI): Wynn Marketing; 1999.
[9] O'Connor FG, Wilder RP. Evaluation of the injured runner. J Back Musculoskeletal Rehabil 1995;5:281–94.
[10] Messier SP, Davis SE, Curl WW, et al. Etiologic factors associated with patellofemoral pain in runners. Med Sci Sports Exerc 1991;23(9):1008–15.
[11] Doxey GE. Assessing quadriceps femoris muscle bulk with girth measurements in subjects with patellofemoral pain. J Orthop Sports Phys Ther 1987;9(5):177–83.
[12] Cowan DN, Jones BH, Robinson JR. Foot morphologic characteristics and risk of exercise-related injury. Arch Fam Med 1993;2(7):773–7.
[13] Bennett JE, Reinking MF, Pluemer B, et al. Factors contributing to the development of medial tibial stress syndrome in high school runners. J Orthop Sports Phys Ther 2001;31(9): 504–10.

[14] Stefanyshyn DJ, Nigg BM. Mechanical energy contribution of the metatarsophalangeal joint to running and sprinting. Journal of Biomechanics 2001;30(11–12):1081–5.

[15] Zeller BL, McCrory JL, Kibler WB, et al. Differences in kinematics and electromyographic activity between men and women during the single-legged squat. Am J Sports Med 2003; 31(3):449–56.

[16] Olmsted LC, Carcia CR, Hertel J, et al. Efficacy of the Star Excursion Balance Tests in detecting reach deficits in subjects with chronic ankle instability. J Athl Train 2002;37(4): 501–6.

[17] Fredericson M, Cookingham CL, Chaudhari AM, et al. Hip abductor weakness in distance runners with iliotibial band syndrome. Clin J Sport Med 2000;10(3):169–75.

[18] Crossley K, Cowan SM, Bennell KL, et al. Patellar taping: is clinical success supported by scientific evidence? Man Ther 2000;5(3):142–50.

[19] Brukner P, Khan K, Agosta J. Foot pain. In: Brukner P, Khan K, editors. Clinical sports medicine. 2nd edition. Sydney (Australia): McGraw-Hill; 2001. p. 584–601.

[20] Fredericson M. Common injuries in runners. Diagnosis, rehabilitation and prevention. Sports Med 1996;21(1):49–72.

[21] Hreljac A, Marshall RN, Hume PA. Evaluation of lower extremity overuse injury potential in runners. Med Sci Sports Exerc 2000;32(9):1635–41.

[22] Hreljac A. Impact and overuse injuries in runners. Med Sci Sports Exercise 2004;36(5):845–9.

[23] Brukner P, Khan K. Biomechanics of common sporting injuries. In: Brukner P, Khan K, editors. Clinical sports medicine. Sydney (Australia): McGraw-Hill; 2001. p. 56–8.

[24] Kibler WB, Goldberg C, Chandler TJ. Functional biomechanical deficits in running athletes with plantar fasciitis. Am J Sports Med 1991;19(1):66–71.

[25] Dreyfuss P, Michaelsen M, Pauza K, et al. The value of medical history and physical examination in diagnosing sacroiliac joint pain. Spine 1996;21(22):2594–602.

[26] Magee DJ. Orthopedic physical assessment. 3rd edition. Philadelphia: WB Saunders Company; 1997.

[27] Crossley K, Bennell K, Green S, et al. Physical therapy for patellofemoral pain. Am J Sports Med 2002;30(6):857–65.

[28] Kendall F, McCreary E, Provance P. Muscles testing and function. 4th edition. Baltimore (MD): Williams and Wilkins; 1993.

[29] Davids JR, Benfanti P, Blackhurst DW, et al. Assessment of femoral anteversion in children with cerebral palsy: accuracy of the trochanteric prominence angle test. J Pediatr Orthop 2002;22(2):173–8.

[30] Cook SD, Brinker MR, Poche M. Running shoes: their relationship to running injuries. Sports Med 1990;10(1):1–8.

[31] Hreljac A. Impact and overuse injuries in runners. Med Sci Sports Exerc 2004;36(5):845–9.

ELSEVIER
SAUNDERS

Phys Med Rehabil Clin N Am
16 (2005) 651–667

PHYSICAL MEDICINE
AND REHABILITATION
CLINICS OF
NORTH AMERICA

# Etiology, Prevention, and Early Intervention of Overuse Injuries in Runners: a Biomechanical Perspective

Alan Hreljac, PhD

*Kinesiology and Health Science Department, California State University, Sacramento,
6000 J Street, Sacramento, CA 95819-6073, USA*

Runners sustain injuries at an alarming rate. According to various epidemiologic studies [1–7], between 27% and 70% of recreational and competitive distance runners can expect to be injured during any 1-year period. The wide range in the results of these epidemiologic studies may be attributed, in part, to differences in the definitions of the terms "runner" and "injury" [8]. Typically, a "runner" has been defined as a person who runs a minimum distance per week (20–30 km is cited often) on a regular basis, and has been running consistently for some minimum period of time (1 to 3 years is cited typically). The definition of "injury" also varies between studies; however, a common definition for a running injury is a musculoskeletal ailment that is attributed to running that causes a restriction of running speed, distance, duration, or frequency for at least 1 week [3,4,9,10].

The most common site of running injuries is the knee. In a recent clinical study [11], an analysis of data from more than 2000 patients who attributed their injuries to running, revealed that approximately 42% of the injuries occurred at the knee. Although the incidence of specific knee injuries that were cited varies slightly, other studies also determined that knee injuries make up close to half of all running injuries that are reported [5,12,13]. The foot, ankle, and lower leg make up almost 40% of the remaining injuries that are reported by these researchers, whereas less than 20% of the running injuries reported occur above the knee. This suggests that there may be some common mechanisms in the etiology of running injuries.

Runners do sustain some acute injuries, such as ankle sprains and fractures, but most running injuries could be classified as "overuse" injuries. An overuse injury has been defined as an injury of the musculoskeletal system

---

*E-mail address:* ahreljac@csus.edu

1047-9651/05/$ - see front matter © 2005 Elsevier Inc. All rights reserved.
doi:10.1016/j.pmr.2005.02.002

that results from the combined fatigue effect over a period of time beyond the capabilities of the specific structure that has been stressed [14,15]. These injuries occur when several repetitive forces are applied to a structure (eg, muscle or tendon); each is less than the acute injury threshold of the structure. The most common overuse injury that is attributed to running is patellofemoral pain syndrome [11,12,13,16]. Other common overuse running injuries include stress fractures, medial tibial stress (shin splints), patellar tendinitis, plantar fasciitis, and Achilles tendinitis [5,11,12].

Although repeated stresses on various structures of the musculoskeletal system often result in an overuse injury, this does not imply that stresses to the musculoskeletal system should be minimized to avoid injury. All biologic structures, such as muscles, tendons, ligaments, and bones, could adapt positively and negatively to the level of stress that is placed upon them. This phenomenon, which was recognized more than 100 years ago [17], articulates that repeated applied stresses that are less than the tensile limit of a structure will lead to positive remodeling, provided that there is an adequate time period between stress applications, whereas any single stress beyond the tensile limit, or repeated stresses that are less than the tensile limit with insufficient time period between stress applications ultimately will lead to an injury [14,15,18].

A stress-frequency curve illustrates how the amount of stress applied to a structure and the number of repetitions of the applied stress are related to injury potential of a particular structure. The theoretic stress-frequency curve (Fig. 1) depicts a simple situation of a load being applied to a structure at regular intervals. The structure represented could be a joint, muscle, bone, or any other structure of the musculoskeletal system that is subjected to stress. The exact limits of stress or frequency would be different for each specific structure, but the stress-frequency curves of each would share a characteristic shape, and convey similar information. Injury would result when the structure is subjected to a stress/frequency combination that is in

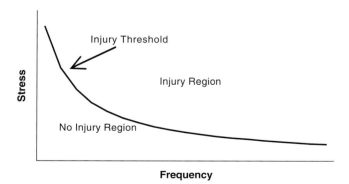

Fig. 1. Effect on overuse injury occurrence due to the theoretical relationship between stress application and frequency.

the "injury region" of the graph (above, and to the right of the curve), whereas injury would be avoided in situations in which the stress/frequency combination falls within the "no injury region" of the graph (below and to the left of the theoretic curve).

This simplistic looking graph (see Fig. 1) gives the impression that predicting an overuse injury should be an easy and straightforward procedure. Rather than being a two-dimensional curve, a true stress-frequency relationship for any given structure is multidimensional, with stresses being applied in all directions, and from a variety of sources (external and internal). In addition, there are multiple structures at each joint (and in each segment) to which stresses are applied; this makes it difficult to estimate the exact level of stress that is placed upon any single structure. To complicate the situation further, a true stress-frequency relationship is not static, but dynamic. When applied stresses are maintained at low levels or removed completely, which happens in several situations, such as prolonged bed rest [19,20] or space flight [21,22], tissue resorption generally occurs. This weakens the structure, shifts the stress-frequency curve downward and to the left, and increases the area of the injury portion of the graph. Conversely, when applied stresses are maintained close to the theoretic curve, but still in the noninjury portion of the graph, positive tissue remodeling likely would occur. This strengthens the structure, shifts the stress-frequency curve upward and to the right, and increases the area of the noninjury portion of the graph.

Not only is the vertical axis of this theoretic relationship more complex than it first appears to be, the horizontal axis (frequency) also has multiple aspects to it. The "frequency" actually can refer to the number of repetitions of an applied stress, the time between each repetition, or the time period between sets of stress applications. All of these aspects of frequency are relevant in a running situation. The number of repetitions of an applied stress is related to the distance traveled or the number of steps taken by a runner. The time between each repetition is related to running speed or stride frequency, and the time period between sets of stress applications is associated with the rest period that is taken between runs, or the number of weekly runs.

## Forces on the body during running

External and internal stresses are applied to the musculoskeletal system during running. The external stresses (forces) that act on the body during running include air resistance, gravity, and ground reaction forces (GRFs). The GRF is the only one of these forces that is likely to contribute to running injuries. When studying gait, GRFs generally are measured by a floor-mounted force platform, and are resolved into their three component directions (anterio–posterior, medio–lateral, and vertical). Internal forces, which include muscle and tendon forces, act upon specific structures of the musculoskeletal system (eg, joints) and also may contribute to running injuries. Because direct measurements of internal forces can only be done invasively, these forces generally are estimated indirectly in a noninvasive manner using an inverse dynamics approach. This approach uses a combination of kinetic, anthropometric, and kinematic data to estimate the forces and torques at joints. With the addition of electromyographic data, various simulation models have been developed that estimate forces that are generated by specific muscles.

Most distance runners are heelstrikers and make first ground contact with the posterior third of the foot [23,24]. This running style produces characteristic GRF-time curves in the anterio–posterior and vertical directions. The anterio–posterior GRF-time curve generally is biphasic. A braking force is apparent for most subjects during approximately the first half of stance. This is followed by a propulsive force of similar magnitude for the remainder of the stance period (Fig. 2). The magnitude of these forces are somewhat speed dependent, but typically are in the range of 0.3 to 0.6 body weights [25].

The vertical GRF-time curve of heelstrike runners generally exhibits two distinctive peaks (Fig. 3). The earlier peak often is referred to as the impact force peak and occurs within the first 10% of the stance period. The magnitude and rate of change (loading rate) of the impact force during running is determined by what a runner does before contact with the ground. Depending upon speed and landing geometry, the vertical impact force peak varies in magnitude from about 1.2 to 3.5 body weights [26,27]. Because this portion of the vertical GRF curve has a brief duration (<30

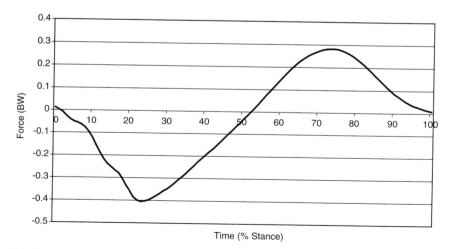

Fig. 2. Representative curve of the anterio–posterior ground reaction force during the stance phase of running. BW, body weights.

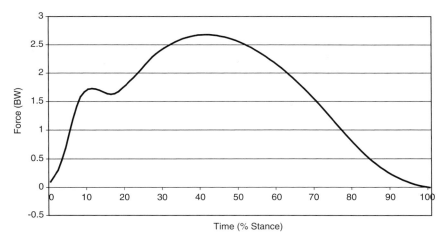

Fig. 3. Representative curve of the vertical ground reaction force during the stance phase of running. BW, body weights.

milliseconds), it is considered to be the high-frequency component of the GRF. Several variables have an effect on impact forces, including the foot and body center of mass velocity at contact, the effective mass of the body at contact (which is influenced by body geometry), the area of contact, and the material properties of the damping elements (eg, soft tissue, shoes, and the surface of contact) [28–30]. The second vertical force peak generally is referred to as the active peak, and occurs at approximately midstance. Active forces take place over the latter 60% to 75% of the stance period, and are considered to be the low-frequency component of the vertical GRF and last up to 200 milliseconds, depending upon speed. Active forces are determined primarily by the movement of a runner during foot contact [31]. Although impact forces have been implicated most often in overuse running injuries [9,32,33], some research exists which suggests that active forces also may play a significant role in a variety of overuse running injuries [34].

GRF-time curves in the medio–lateral direction are variable and have low magnitudes. Primarily for these reasons, medio–lateral forces have been ignored by most researchers when investigating the causes of running injuries. In recent studies, however, the contribution of the medio–lateral forces to varus and valgus moments have been examined [32]. Although it has yet to be determined, it is possible that the medio–lateral forces do contribute to a variety of overuse running injuries.

## Etiology of running injuries

Despite the great deal of literature that has been dedicated to the subject of running injuries, comparatively little empiric evidence exists concerning the causes of these injuries. Many of the articles that have been written regarding the etiology of running injuries are speculative in nature. Several researchers who have conducted biomechanical studies that used only healthy subjects have made conclusions regarding the possible effect of various factors on running injuries, even though no evidence exists to suggest that the factors in question are risk factors for running injuries. Many other articles have been written by health care providers who have treated several people who had injuries that were attributed to running. Generally, using sound reasoning (as done by the biomechanists), along with survey data (but little experimental evidence), these researchers have attempted to identify risk factors that are associated with various overuse running injuries. Scientific research has not been able to verify or refute most of the speculations that were made in these retrospective clinical studies. All that can be stated with certainty is that the etiology of overuse running injuries is multifactorial and diverse [5,18,35].

The variables that have been identified as risk factors for overuse running injuries vary slightly from study to study, but they can be placed into three general categories, including training, anatomic, and bio-mechanical factors. Although it occasionally has been suggested that particular running injuries or sites of injuries are associated with specific risk factors, current scientific research has yet to reach the point of being able to distinguish between the causes of specific running injuries, nor is it likely that exact mechanisms for specific injuries ever will be determined. Some researchers concluded that no anatomic or biomechanical factor correlates with a specific type of injury in a reliable fashion [36,37]. There are, however, several risk factors that may be associated with a variety of running injuries. In the subsequent discussion of these factors, "running injuries" often have been grouped together, rather than being examined specifically.

The training variables (errors) that have been identified most often as risk factors for running injuries include excessive running distance, too high of a training intensity, and rapid increases in weekly running distance or intensity [2,5,36–40]. The general mechanism by which each of these training errors could lead to overuse injuries may be understood by the examining how these variables affect the stress-frequency relationship. Running a greater distance without an increase in running speed obviously increases the number of repetitions of the applied stress because the number of steps taken is increased. Thus, running an excessive distance places the various musculoskeletal structures of a runner further to the right on the stress-frequency curve and increases the possibility that one or more structures enter the injury region of the graph. A high-intensity running program relates to running at faster speeds. Faster running generally produces greater GRFs, as well as greater stresses on bones, joints, muscles, and tendons [26,41,42]. This places all of these structures higher on the stress-frequency graph and increases the likelihood of injury.

Rapid changes in distance or intensity are more complex to explain by the stress-frequency relationship. When a structure is subjected to a stress-frequency combination that is close to the stress-frequency curve, yet below and to the left of the curve, positive remodeling of the structure may shift the curve upward and to the right. Increases in distance or intensity (or both) may place the structure further upward and to the right on the stress-frequency curve. If increases in running distance and intensity (frequency and stress) are gradual, it is possible for the upward and right shifting of the stress-frequency curve that is due to positive remodeling to outpace the upward and right direction movement that is due to increases in distance and intensity. But, rapid increases in distance or intensity may cause the structure to cross the curve from the noninjury region to the injury region, even when some positive remodeling and shifting of the curve has occurred.

Two related training variables also have been implicated as risk factors in running injuries—the surface and shoes that are chosen for training [43–45]. It was suggested that running with worn-out shoes or on harder (less compliant) running surfaces may produce greater stresses on the body [30,46,47], and therefore, are risk factors for injury. These variables, however, are examples for which there is a lack of empiric evidence to link them with overuse running injuries, even though there are logical reasons to speculate that they are associated with these injuries. It is possible that these factors may be determined to be true risk factors for running injuries, but at the present time, the association between these factors and overuse running injuries is purely conjecture.

Performing stretching exercises before running is another training-related variable that has been examined as a possible risk factor for running injuries. There have been conflicting conclusions drawn regarding the association of this factor with overuse running injuries. Although several researchers reported that people who stretch regularly before running experience a greater injury rate than those who do not stretch regularly [2,6,48], others did not find an association between stretching before running and injuries [4,9,49]. No empiric study has reported that regular stretching before running reduces the number of running injuries, even though this practice has been advocated as a means of preventing running injuries [50]. Data that are related to the stretching and warm-up habits of runners generally rely upon surveys or self reporting; therefore, these results must be considered cautiously. It is possible that stretching before running is important for some runners, whereas it may not be necessary for others.

Several clinical studies have estimated that more than 60% of running injuries could be attributed to training error [3,12,37,38,51]. Pragmatically, it could be stated that, in actual fact, all overuse running injuries are the result of training errors. To sustain an overuse injury, a runner must have subjected some musculoskeletal structure to a stress-frequency combination that crossed over to the right and above the current stress-frequency curve (into the injury region) for that specific structure. This is accomplished only when an individual makes an error in his/her training program by exceeding his/her current limit of running distance or intensity in such a way that the negative remodeling of the injured structure predominated over the repair process as a result of the stresses that are placed on the structure. It is obvious that the location of the stress-frequency curve for a given structure varies from structure to structure, and from individual to individual; however, there is no doubt that every overuse injury that is sustained by runners could have been avoided by training differently based upon individual limitations, or in some cases, by not training at all. There are some people who should be advised (correctly) against running as a form of exercise because the risk for injury would be excessive merely because of participation.

The idea that all overuse running injuries are a result of training errors is appealing from a medical practitioner's viewpoint. Obviously, training variables are factors over which a runner has control; therefore, advice regarding training methods could be given easily. By correctly determining the specific aspects of an individual's training program that had been producing deleterious effects, a medical practitioner would be able to advise a runner properly regarding how to modify his/her training program to minimize the chance of a subsequent injury. Knowledge of the training variables that are associated with overuse running injuries has a great clinical value, but this knowledge does not allow a scientist to understand the mechanisms that lead to an overuse running injury.

With most, if not all, overuse injuries, there must exist some underlying anatomic or biomechanical factors that would prevent one runner from training for as long, as often, or as intensely as another runner before incurring an overuse injury. Stated in another way, the question could be asked "Why does each individual runner (and each individual musculoskeletal structure) have a different injury threshold?". It is conceivable that two individuals who have comparable anatomic and stride characteristics train together, but only one of the individuals sustains an overuse injury. In this case, and in most cases of overuse running injuries, it is logical to hypothesize that some anatomic or biomechanical variations between individuals could account for differences in injury susceptibility.

Abnormalities or variations in anatomic or anthropometric variables may place an individual at an increased risk for an overuse running injury. Even if the level of external biomechanical stresses (GRFs) that is applied to the body is within a "normal" range, anthropometric variations between individuals may result in increased amounts of internal stresses applied to various musculoskeletal structures. This would affect an individual's tolerance level to injury in terms of distance, intensity, and frequency. Generally, these anthropometric variables are not within the control of a runner or medical practitioner, but some variables can be modified or manipulated with appropriate interventions.

Anthropometric variables that have been implicated as causes of overuse running injuries include high longitudinal arches (pes cavus), ankle range of motion, leg length discrepancies, and lower extremity alignment abnormalities. There is no consensus among researchers, however, regarding the effect of most of these variables on overuse running injuries based upon the conflicting results that are reported in the literature. Pes cavus has been implicated as a risk factor for running injuries, according to several studies [39,44,52,53], but others concluded that arch height is not a risk factor in running injuries [54–57].

The relationship between ankle flexibility and overuse running injuries is even more controversial. Runners who had a greater sagittal plane ankle range of motion were determined to be at greater risk for overuse injuries than runners who had less ankle mobility, according to some researchers [37,39,53]. Other studies reported that sagittal plane ankle range of motion does not differ significantly between groups of runners who had sustained lower extremity injuries and groups of uninjured control subjects [9,50]. Still, one other study disagreed with both of these possibilities, and concluded that reduced ankle flexibility is a risk factor in overuse running injuries [54]. This study was based upon an examination of military recruits who sustained stress fractures during training. The recruits who sustained stress fractures tended to have less ankle flexibility than recruits who did not sustain these injuries.

There also is controversy regarding anthropometric variables that could be grouped together as lower extremity alignment abnormalities, such as leg length discrepancies and excessive Q-angle. These variables were shown to be associated with overuse running injuries by some investigators [3,15,38], although others determined that lower extremity alignment abnormalities are not associated with an increased risk for overuse injuries in runners [54–57].

Some of the discrepancies in studies that search for a link between anthropometric variables and running injuries may be due to differences in experimental methodology (measuring techniques), and in the definition of the various anthropometric abnormalities that were analyzed. In addition, it is likely that people who possess severe abnormalities could not have participated in many of the studies because of the protocols that generally included people who were engaged in running activities at the time of the study. It is possible that people who had severe problems realized that running is an activity in which they could not participate safely. Another reason for discrepancies in these studies may be the fact that anthropometric variables must act in combination with biomechanical factors to produce an injury. These biomechanical variables often differ significantly between subjects.

It is possible that a runner who has an identified anthropometric risk factor exhibits "favorable" biomechanical conditions that could allow the runner to avoid injury. Similarly, in a situation in which all anthropometric variables are similar between subjects, variations in biomechanical variables may result in an overuse injury to one individual and not another. Several early biomechanical studies speculated that a link exists between various biomechanical variables and overuse running injuries [30,43,58–60]. Most of these biomechanical factors could be classified as kinetic or rearfoot kinematic variables. The mechanism whereby kinetic variables increase the risk for an overuse injury is obvious. Abnormally large external or internal stresses on the musculoskeletal system could shift a specific structure into the injury portion of a stress-frequency curve. It is generally believed that rearfoot kinematic variables that are outside of the physiologically "normal" range may redistribute forces in such a manner that a particularly vulnerable structure would be affected.

Among the kinetic variables that have been speculated to be a cause of overuse running injuries are the magnitude of impact forces [58], the rate of impact loading [24], the magnitude of active (propulsive) forces [60], and the magnitude of knee joint forces and moments [59]. The assumption that these kinetic variables lead to overuse injuries generally has been based upon theoretic models and sound reasoning; however, until recently, there has been little experimental verification of these speculations. In a study in which female subjects who had a history of stress fractures were compared with a control group of uninjured subjects, the injured subjects were exhibited greater peak vertical impact GRFs, impact loading rates, and peak tibial accelerations [32]. Similar results that were reported by Grimston et al [33] found that female runners who had experienced stress fractures produced significantly greater vertical impact forces than subjects who did not have stress fractures. These results were in agreement with another recent study in which previously injured runners (men and women) were compared with runners who had never sustained an overuse injury [9]. The investigators reported that the group of previously injured runners exhibited greater vertical impact forces and loading rates than the uninjured runners. In a study that used similar methodology, it was reported that runners who developed patellofemoral pain syndrome displayed greater active vertical forces than uninjured control subjects [34]. Although no other studies have found vertical active (propulsive) forces to be a risk factor for overuse running injuries, many researchers who have studied the contribution of kinetic variables to overuse running injuries have not reported active forces in their studies. Therefore, it is possible that this variable may be a risk factor that has not been examined extensively.

Injury risk may differ between subjects, even when external kinetic variables are similar. One possible explanation of this phenomenon is that slight (and possibly undetected) anatomic variations between people could result in differences in internal joint kinetics. To estimate these forces and moments noninvasively, the technique of inverse dynamics is used. Until recently, this technique had not been applied to research that was related to running injuries. In a study that compared a group of runners who had suffered from patellofemoral pain syndrome with a group of control subjects, increased knee joint forces and moments were a contributing factor in the development of patellofemoral pain syndrome in runners [61].

The rearfoot kinematic variables that have been suggested most often to be associated with overuse running injuries are the magnitude and rate of foot pronation. Excessive pronation was implicated as a contributing factor to overuse running injuries in several clinical studies and reviews of overuse running injuries [18,34,36–38,43,44,62]. In many of these studies, a static evaluation of pronation was conducted on injured runners; the results suggested that injured runners often were overpronators. The little experimental evidence that exists in relation to these parameters is conflicting. One study that partially supported the speculation of these clinical studies, reported that groups of injured runners exhibited greater maximum pronation angles and had greater maximum pronation velocities than a group of uninjured control subjects [39]. The results were most evident in the group of subjects who suffered from shin splints. Similar results were reported in a comparison between shin splint sufferers and uninjured control subjects during barefoot running [63]. Contradictory results were found in a more recent study which found that runners who had never sustained an overuse injury exhibited a greater pronation velocity than runners who had sustained an overuse injury previously [9]. Another study that compared runners who suffered from patellofemoral pain syndrome with a group of uninjured control subjects found no differences in any rearfoot variable between groups [34].

The effect that a particular level of impact force has on a body during running is related to the amount and rate of pronation. Pronation is a protective mechanism during running because it allows impact forces to be attenuated over a longer period of time than would occur without pronation. For this reason, some researchers have suggested that it is conceivable that a higher level of pronation is favorable during running, provided that it falls within "normal" physiologic limitations, and that it does not continue beyond midstance [9,64]. After midstance, it is necessary for the foot to become more rigid in preparation for toe-off. In a recent review of overuse injuries in runners, Hreljac [65] concluded that "runners who have developed stride patterns which incorporate relatively low levels of impact forces, and a moderately rapid rate of pronation are at a reduced risk for incurring overuse running injuries." Severe overpronators may be at an increased risk for injury because of the potentially large torques that are generated, and the potential instability that is associated with running in this style.

## Early intervention

Although a retrospective treatment of running injuries may assist runners to heal following an overuse injury, a preferable approach to the problem would be to act proactively. A proactive approach could take many forms, such as the education of current and prospective runners regarding a sensible approach to training; proper fitting and selection of shoes; and the establishment of a screening process whereby medical practitioners could identify runners who are at high risk for overuse injuries, and advise these runners accordingly.

For a screening process to have widespread appeal, it must be simple to administer and it must be reliable. No such screening process is available for running injuries assessment; however, some researchers have taken the first steps in the establishment of such a screening process. Studies are underway in which researchers are attempting to establish whether a combination of anthropometric and biomechanical factors could be used to predict the occurrence of an overuse running injury [65]. Even if these studies are successful, however, they would have limited usefulness because the screening tests would require a researcher or clinician to take several anthropometric measurements and conduct a series of biomechanical tests. Because of the limited availability of biomechanical testing facilities, and the need for trained personnel, this type of screening process realistically could not become widespread. But, assuming that a small number of anthropometric and biomechanical parameters that are associated with overuse running injuries could be identified, follow-up studies could be conducted that would attempt to find easily measurable variables that are correlated highly with these variables. If this can be established, then the widespread screening of runners and prospective runners could become realistic. Currently, that goal is not within reach.

One intervention that is within reach of most runners is the proper selection of running shoes. Running shoes are the only pieces of protective equipment that are worn by a runner, and as such, it is critical that a runner chooses shoes wisely. The number of running shoe choices that is available might be overwhelming to some people [66]. Because it has been suggested that low levels of impact forces and a moderately rapid rate of pronation are stride characteristics that appear to reduce the risk for incurring overuse running injuries [65], it follows that an ideal pair of running shoes minimizes impact forces and provides stability while allowing the foot to pronate naturally.

One running shoe design parameter that has an effect on cushioning and stability properties of a shoe is the midsole density (hardness). Although material tests on shoes consistently demonstrate that softer-soled shoes attenuate forces to a greater extent than harder shoes when subjected to an impact tester, there have been conflicting reports regarding the effects of varying the midsole density on cushioning and stability parameters during subject tests [67]. Although some researchers found that subject tests agree with the results of material tests regarding cushioning variables, with shoes that have softer midsoles producing lower initial vertical GRFs [68], others reported that softer shoes produced greater initial vertical GRFs than harder shoes [69–72]. Still others have reported that there are no differences between soft and hard shoes in terms of impact forces [43,73]. Conflicting results also have been reported in variables that are believed to be indicative of stability characteristics. Some researchers found that softer shoes allow greater amounts and rates of pronation than harder shoes [43,74], whereas others reported the opposite [71]. Still others have concluded that there are no differences in the amount of pronation that is allowed by softer or harder shoes [47].

In an attempt to review the available data objectively, Hreljac and Marshall [75] conducted a meta-analysis of the existing literature. They determined that shoes with harder midsoles reduce the initial impact forces while allowing greater rearfoot movement during the initial ground contact phase. They also noted that there was a large amount of variability between subjects and between studies, which indicated that individuals respond uniquely to changes in midsole hardness. Thus, the "proper" selection of running shoes would require an individual runner to conduct biomechanical tests on several running shoes to determine which shoe best attenuated impact forces while allowing a reasonable amount and rate of pronation. This could only be done in a limited number of facilities, so it is not a feasible alternative.

Although conducting a series of biomechanical tests on several shoes would be preferable, the selection of running shoes for any individual could be based upon two simple guidelines. It was suggested that the most important criteria in the selection of running shoes are fit [66] and comfort [76,77]. Running shoes that meet these criteria are likely to provide optimal levels of cushioning and stability.

In the absence of a simple screening process, the education of current and prospective runners probably is the most feasible approach to proactively prevent running injuries. Besides being informed of the simple criteria that could be followed in selecting running shoes, runners should be taught how to incorporate sensible training habits into their schedules. It may not be possible or practical to teach people to run with a stride that incorporates lower impact forces and moderate rates of pronation, but there are training habits that runners could adopt which reduce impact forces and minimize the effects of these forces on the body. Among the advice that should be given to, and followed by, runners who are at risk for sustaining an overuse running injury, is to reduce training speed as a means of reducing impact forces. It was concluded in several studies that impact forces increase as speed increases [26,27,41,78]. Sufficiently long rest periods should be encouraged to assure that positive remodeling is able to occur between training sessions. A guideline for increasing weekly running distance that has been suggested often is that runners should not increase running distance by more than 10% per week [35,36,38,49]. The same suggestion likely would apply to intensity of training. A sensible suggestion for runners who have sustained repeated injuries would be to reduce the distance run during each session, and overall weekly distance. But, as pointed out by Marti et al [5], it probably would be as difficult to motivate determined runners to reduce running distance as it would be to motivate sedentary people to take up running as an activity.

664 HRELJAC

# References

[1] Caspersen CJ, Powell KE, Koplan JP, et al. The incidence of injuries and hazards in recreational and fitness runners. Med Sci Sports Exerc 1984;16:113–4.

[2] Jacobs SJ, Berson BL. Injuries to runners: a study of entrants to a 10,000 meter race. Am J Sports Med 1986;14:151–5.

[3] Lysholm J, Wiklander J. Injuries in runners. Am J Sports Med 1987;15:168–71.

[4] Macera CA, Pate RR, Powell KE, et al. Predicting lower-extremity injuries among habitual runners. Arch Intern Med 1989;149:2565–8.

[5] Marti B, Vader JP, Minder CE, et al. On the epidemiology of running injuries: The 1984 Bern Grand-Prix Study. Am J Sports Med 1988;16:285–93.

[6] Rochcongar P, Pernes J, Carre F, et al. Occurrence of running injuries: a survey among 1153 runners. Sci Sports 1995;10:15–9.

[7] Walter SD, Hart LE, McIntosh JM, et al. The Ontario Cohort Study of running-related injuries. Arch Intern Med 1989;149:2561–4.

[8] Hoeberigs JH. Factors related to the incidence of running injuries: a review. Sports Med 1992;13:408–22.

[9] Hreljac A, Marshall RN, Hume PA. Evaluation of lower extremity overuse injury potential in runners. Med Sci Sports Exerc 2000;32:1635–41.

[10] Koplan JP, Powell KE, Sikes RK, et al. The risk of exercise: an epidemiological study of the benefits and risks of running. JAMA 1982;248:3118–21.

[11] Taunton JE, Ryan MB, Clement DB, et al. A retrospective case-control analysis of 2002 running injuries. Br J Sports Med 2002;36(2):95–101.

[12] Clement DB, Taunton JE, Smart GW, et al. A survey of overuse running injuries. Physician Sports Med 1981;9(5):47–58.

[13] Pinshaw R, Atlas V, Noakes T. The nature and response to therapy of 196 consecutive injuries seen at a runners' clinic. S Afr Med J 1984;65:291–8.

[14] Elliott BC. Adolescent overuse sporting injuries: a biomechanical review. Australian Sports Commission Program 1990;23:1–9.

[15] Stanish WD. Overuse injuries in athletes: a perspective. Med Sci Sports Exerc 1984;16:1–7.

[16] Ballas M, Tylko J, Cookson D. Common overuse running injuries: diagnosis and management. Am Fam Physician 1997;55:2473–80.

[17] Wolff J. Das gesetz der transformation der knochen [The law of bone remodeling]. Berlin: Hirschwald; 1892 [in German].

[18] Rolf C. Overuse injuries of the lower extremity in runners. Scand J Med Sci Sports 1995;5:181–90.

[19] Inoue M, Tanaka H, Moriwake T, et al. Altered biochemical markers of bone turnover in humans during 120 days of bed rest. Bone 2000;26(3):281–6.

[20] LeBlanc AD, Schneider VS, Evans HJ, et al. Bone mineral loss and recovery after 17 weeks of bed rest. J Bone Min Res 1990;5(8):843–50.

[21] Lang T, LeBlanc A, Evans H, et al. Cortical and trabecular bone mineral loss from the spine and hip in long-duration spaceflight. J Bone Min Res 2004;19(6):1006–14.

[22] Vico L, Collet P, Guignandon A, et al. Effects of long-term microgravity exposure on cancellous and cortical weight-bearing bones of cosmonauts. Lancet 2000;355:1607–11.

[23] Bates BT, Osternig LR, Mason B, et al. Lower extremity function during the support phase of running. In: Asmussen E, Jorgensen K, editors. Biomechanics VI-A. Baltimore (MD): University Park; 1978. p. 30–9.

[24] Nigg BM, Denoth J, Neukomm PA. Quantifying the load on the human body: problems and some possible solutions. In: Morecki A, Fidelus K, Kedzior K, et al, editors. Biomechanics VII-B. Baltimore (MD): University Park; 1981. p. 88–99.

[25] Diss CE. The reliability of kinetic and kinematic variables used to analyze normal gait. Gait Posture 2001;14:98–103.

[26] Keller TS, Weisberger AM, Ray JL, et al. Relationship between vertical ground reaction force and speed during walking, slow jogging, and running. Clin Biomech (Bristol, Avon) 1996;11(5):253–9.

[27] Ricard MD, Veatch S. Effect of running speed and aerobic dance jump height on vertical ground reaction forces. J Appl Biomech 1994;10:14–27.

[28] Derrick TR, Caldwell GE, Hamill J. Modeling the stiffness characteristics of the human body while running with various stride lengths. J Appl Biomech 2000;16(1):36–51.

[29] Gerritsen KGM, van den Bogert AJ, Nigg BM. Direct dynamics simulation of the impact phase in heel-toe running. J Biomech 1995;28:661–8.

[30] Nigg BM. Biomechanical aspects of running. In: Nigg BM, editor. Biomechanics of running shoes. Champaign (IL): Human Kinetics; 1986. p. 1–25.

[31] Nigg BM. External force measurements with sport shoes and playing surfaces. In: Nigg BM, Kerr BA, editors. Biomechanical aspects of sport shoes and playing surfaces. Calgary (Canada): University Press; 1983. p. 11–23.

[32] Ferber R, McClay-Davis I, Hamill J, et al. Kinetic variables in subjects with previous lower extremity stress fractures. Med Sci Sports Exerc 2002;34:S5.

[33] Grimston SK, Nigg BM, Fisher V, et al. External loads throughout a 45 minute run in stress fracture and non-stress fracture runners. Proceedings of the 14th ISB Congress. Paris: International Society of Biomechanics; 1993. p. 512–3.

[34] Messier SP, Davis SE, Curl WW, et al. Etiologic factors associated with patellofemoral pain in runners. Med Sci Sports Exerc 1991;23:1008–15.

[35] van Mechelen W. Can running injuries be effectively prevented? Sports Med 1995;19:161–5.

[36] James SL. Running injuries of the knee. AAOS Instr Course Lect 1998;47:407–17.

[37] James SL, Jones DC. Biomechanical aspects of distance running injuries. In: Cavanagh PR, editor. Biomechanics of distance running. Champaign (IL): Human Kinetics; 1990. p. 249–69.

[38] James SL, Bates BT, Osternig LR. Injuries to runners. Am J Sports Med 1978;6:40–50.

[39] Messier SP, Pittala KA. Etiologic factors associated with selected running injuries. Med Sci Sports Exerc 1988;20:501–5.

[40] Paty JG Jr. Running injuries. Curr Opin Rheumatol 1994;6:203–9.

[41] Hamill J, Bates BT, Sawhill JA, et al. Comparisons between selected ground reaction force parameters at different running speeds. Med Sci Sports Exerc 1982;14:143.

[42] Mercer JA, Vance J, Hreljac A, et al. Relationship between shock attenuation and stride length during running at different velocities. Eur J Appl Physiol 2002;87:403–8.

[43] Clarke TE, Frederick EC, Hamill CL. The effects of shoe design parameters on rearfoot control in running. Med Sci Sports Exerc 1983;15:376–81.

[44] McKenzie DC, Clement DB, Taunton JE. Running shoes, orthotics, and injuries. Sports Med 1985;2:334–47.

[45] Robbins SE, Gouw GJ. Athletic footwear and chronic overloading. A brief review. Sports Med 1990;9:76–85.

[46] Frederick EC, Hagy JL. Factors affecting peak vertical ground reaction forces in running. Int J Sports Biomech 1986;2:41–9.

[47] Stacoff A, Denoth J, Kaelin X, et al. Running injuries and shoe construction: some possible relationships. Int J Sports Biomech 1988;4:342–57.

[48] Hart LE, Walter SD, McIntosh JM, et al. The effect of stretching and warmup on the development of musculoskeletal injuries (MSI) in distance runners. Med Sci Sports Exerc 1989;21:S59.

[49] Blair SN, Kohl HW, Goodyear NN. Rates and risks for running and exercise injuries: studies in three populations. Res Q Exerc Sport 1987;58:221–8.

[50] van Mechelen WH, Hlobil H, Kemper HCG, et al. Prevention of running injuries by warm-up, cool-down, and stretching exercises. Am J Sports Med 1993;21:711–9.

[51] Kibler WB. Clinical aspects of muscle injury. Med Sci Sports Exerc 1990;22:450–2.

[52] Cowan D, Jones B, Robinson J. Medial longitudinal arch height and risk of training associated injury. Med Sci Sports Exerc 1989;21:S60.

[53] Warren BL, Jones CJ. Predicting plantar fasciitis in runners. Med Sci Sports Exerc 1987;19: 71–3.

[54] Montgomery LC, Nelson FRT, Norton JP, et al. Orthopedic history and examination in the etiology of overuse injuries. Med Sci Sports Exerc 1989;21:237–43.

[55] Pollard CD, McKeown KA, Ferber R, et al. Selected structural characteristics of female runners with and without lower extremity stress fractures. Med Sci Sports Exerc 2002;34: S177.

[56] Rudzki SJ. Injuries in Australian army recruits. Part II. Location and cause of injuries seen in recruits. Mil Med 1997;162:477–80.

[57] Wen DY, Puffer JC, Schmalzried TP. Lower extremity alignment and risk of overuse injuries in runners. Med Sci Sports Exerc 1997;29:1291–8.

[58] Cavanagh PR, LaFortune MA. Ground reaction forces in distance running. J Biomech 1980; 13:397–406.

[59] Scott SH, Winter DA. Internal forces at chronic running injury sites. Med Sci Sports Exerc 1990;22:357–69.

[60] Winter DA. Moments of force and mechanical power in jogging. J Biomech 1983;16:91–7.

[61] Stefanyshyn DJ, Stergiou P, Lun VMY, et al. Knee joint moments and patellofemoral pain syndrome in runners Part I: A case control study Part II: A prospective cohort study. Presented at the Fourth Symposium on Footwear Biomechanics. Canmore, Alberta, Canada, August 5–9, 1999.

[62] Jones DC. Achilles tendon problems in runners. AAOS Instr Course Lect 1998;47:419–27.

[63] Viitasalo JT, Kvist M. Some biomechanical aspects of the foot and ankle in athletes with and without shin splints. Am J Sports Med 1983;11:125–30.

[64] Subotnick SI. The biomechanics of running: implications for the prevention of foot injuries. Sports Med 1995;2:144–53.

[65] Hreljac A. Impact and overuse injuries in runners. Med Sci Sports Exerc 2004;36:845–9.

[66] Whyatt A. Shoes made simple: a buyer's guide to the biomechanics of sneakers. Women's Sports Fitness 1998;1(9):43–4.

[67] Frederick EC. Biomechanical consequences of sport shoe design. Med Sci Sports Exerc 1987; 19:375–99.

[68] DeVita P, Bates BT. Intraday reliability of ground reaction force data. J Hum Mov Stud 1988;7:73–85.

[69] Cavanagh PR. Current approaches, problems and future directions in shoe evaluation techniques. In: Winter DA, Norman RW, Wells RP, et al, editors. Biomechanics IX-B. Champaign (IL): Human Kinetics; 1985. p. 123–7.

[70] de Koning JJ, Nigg BM. Kinematic factors affecting initial peak vertical ground reaction forces in running. J Biomech 1994;27:673.

[71] Kaelin X, Denoth J, Stacoff A, et al. Cushioning during running-material tests contra subject test. In: Perren S, Schneider E, editors. Biomechanics: current interdisciplinary research. Dordrecht (The Netherlands): Maartinus Nijhoff; 1985. p. 651–6.

[72] Snel JG, Delleman NJ, Heerkens YF, et al. Shock-absorbing characteristics of running shoes during actual running. In: Winter DA, Norman RW, Wells RP, et al, editors. Biomechanics IX-B. Champaign (IL): Human Kinetics; 1985. p. 133–7.

[73] Nigg BM, Bahlsen HA, Lüthi SM, et al. The influence of running velocity and midsole hardness on external impact forces in heel-toe running. J Biomech 1987;20:951–9.

[74] de Wit B, de Clerq D, Lenoir M. The effect of varying midsole hardness on impact forces and foot motion during foot contact in running. J Appl Biomech 1995;11:395–406.

[75] Hreljac A, Marshall RN. The effect of varying midsole hardness on force attenuation and rearfoot movement during running: a meta-analysis. Presented at the Fourth Symposium on Footwear Biomechanics. Canmore, Alberta, Canada, August 5–9, 1999.

[76] Miller JE, Nigg BM, Liu W, et al. Influence of foot, leg and shoe characteristics on subjective comfort. Foot Ankle Int 2000;21:759–67.

[77] Mündermann A, Nigg BM, Stefanyshyn DJ, et al. Development of a reliable method to assess footwear comfort during running. Gait Posture 2002;16:38–45.

[78] Mercer JA, Black D, Branks D, et al. Stride length effects on ground reaction forces during running. Presented at the 25th Annual Meeting of the American Society of Biomechanics. San Diego, August 1–5, 2001.

ELSEVIER
SAUNDERS

Phys Med Rehabil Clin N Am
16 (2005) 669–689

PHYSICAL MEDICINE
AND REHABILITATION
CLINICS OF
NORTH AMERICA

# Muscular Balance, Core Stability, and Injury Prevention for Middle- and Long-Distance Runners

Michael Fredericson, MD[a],*, Tammara Moore, PT[b]

[a]Department of Orthopaedic Surgery,
Division of Physical Medicine and Rehabilitation,
Stanford University School of Medicine,
3000 Pasteur Drive R105B, Stanford, CA 94305, USA
[b]Sports and Orthopedic Leaders Physical Therapy, 5297A College Avenue,
Oakland, CA 94618, USA

Martial artists long have recognized the importance of well-developed core musculature. One of the main differences between a novice practitioner and a black belt is the black belt's development and use of his core (called "center" or "Ki") to produce balanced, powerful, and explosive movements. For middle- and long-distance runners—whose chosen sport involves balanced and powerful movements of the body propelling itself forward and catching itself in complex motor patterns—this stable core, as well as a strong foundation of muscular balance, is essential. In many runners, however—even those at an Olympic level—this core musculature is not developed fully. Weakness or lack of sufficient coordination in core musculature can lead to less efficient movements, compensatory movement patterns, strain, overuse, and injury. This article discusses the importance of muscle balance and core stability for injury prevention and for improving a distance runner's efficiency and performance. It includes a detailed series of core exercises that can be incorporated gradually into a runner's training program. The program starts with restoration of normal muscle length and mobility to correct any muscle imbalances. Next, fundamental lumbo-pelvic stability exercises are introduced which teach the athlete to activate the deeper core musculature. When this has been mastered, advanced lumbo-pelvic stability exercises on the physioball are added for greater challenge. As the athlete transitions to the standing position, sensory motor training is

---

* Corresponding author.
*E-mail address:* mfred2@stanford.edu (M. Fredericson).

---

**Box 1. Common tight and inhibited muscles in runners**

*Postural (tendency to shortness and tightness)*
Gastroc-soleus (predominately soleus)
Rectus femoris
Iliopsoas
Tensor fascia lata
Hamstrings
Short thigh adductors
Quadratus lumborum
Piriformis
Sartorius

*Phasic (tendency to weakness and inhibition)*
Tibialis anterior
Peroneals
Vastus medialis
Long thigh adductors
Gluteus maximus, medius, and minimus

---

used to stimulate the subcortex and provides a basis for functional movement exercises that promote balance, coordination, precision, and skill acquisition. The ultimate goal of core stabilization is to train "movements" and "positions" rather than muscles. Exercises are most effective when they mirror the demands of the athlete's sport.

**The role of the core**

In essence, the "core" can be viewed as a box with the abdominals in the front, paraspinals and gluteals in the back, the diaphragm as the roof, and the pelvic floor and hip girdle musculature as the bottom [1]. Within this box are 29 pairs of muscles that help to stabilize the spine, pelvis, and kinetic chain during functional movements. When the system works efficiently, the result is appropriate distribution of forces; optimal control and efficiency of movement; adequate absorption of ground-impact forces; and an absence of excessive compressive, translation, or shearing forces on the joints of the kinetic chain. This efficiency requires an integration of the myofascial, articular, and neural systems, which, in turn, requires optimal functioning of the muscles, including the muscles' ability to contract in a coordinated manner and with sufficient motor control and neuromodulation so the joints receive adequate compression through the articular structures. This model supports an integrated model of joint function [2] and leads to optimal length-tension ratios and optimal force coupling of the muscles. Addition-

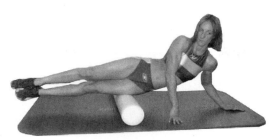

Fig. 1. Foam roll for soft tissue mobilization. The athlete is positioned side-lying with the foam roller just below the hip bone. She then rolls along the outer thigh, from the top of the knee to the bottom of the hip bone. This may be painful, especially at first, so perform in moderation.

ally, this model sets the stage for optimal postural alignment, normal movement patterns, and a minimal potential for joint dysfunction. Biomechanical studies showed clearly that joint dysfunction anywhere from the spine to the feet can lead to compromise elsewhere in the kinetic chain [3].

The first stage in developing a stable core is to develop the abdominal muscles. Richardson and coworkers [1] discovered that there are two different types of muscles fibers (slow-twitch and fast-twitch) that comprise the abdominal muscles; because of this different fiber composition, different exercise regimens are required to train the abdominal muscles properly. Slow-twitch fibers primarily make up the local muscle system—the muscles of the deeper abdominal muscle layers. These muscles are closer to the center of rotation of the spinal segments and, with their shorter muscle lengths, are ideal for controlling intersegmental motion, maintaining mechanical stiffness of the spine, and are best suited to respond to changes in posture and extrinsic loads. The key muscles of this system include the transversus abdominus, multifidi, internal oblique, deep transversospinalis,

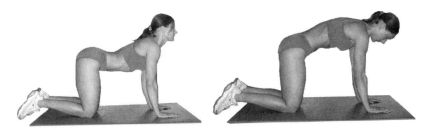

Fig. 2. Cat-Camel exercise. The athlete should lightly brace the abdominal wall. With the hands directly beneath the shoulders and the knees directly beneath the hips, the entire spine is engaged in a synchronous motion, moving in flexion and extension. Correct form requires hip motion to enable proper lumbar function. To help athletes achieve this motion in extension, McGill [4] recommends that the athlete thinks of "sticking the butt out." Six to 10 cycles of this exercise usually are sufficient.

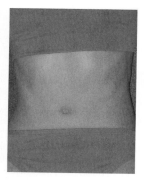

Fig. 3. Abdominal bracing. The abdominal bracing technique involves a submaximal isometric contraction of the three layers of the abdominal wall (rectus, obliques, and transverse) which produces a true muscular girdle around the spine to buttress against buckling and shear instability.

and pelvic floor muscles. McGill [4] described a "hoop" around the abdomen that consists of the abdominal fascia anteriorly, the lumbodorsal fascia posteriorly, and the transverse abdominis and internal obliques muscles laterally. In combination with the intra-abdominal pressure mechanism, activation of this system serves to tension the hoop and provide a stabilizing corset to the spine.

Fast-twitch fibers, conversely, primarily make up the global muscle system (superficial or outer-layer muscles). These muscles possess long levers and large moment arms that are capable of producing large outputs of torque, with an emphasis on speed, power, and larger arcs of movement [5]. The main muscles in this layer are the erector spinae, external oblique, and

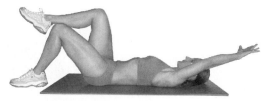

Fig. 4. Supine bent-knee raises. This is a fundamental exercise for recruiting the deep abdominal muscles and for lumbo-pelvic control. The athlete lies on her back, with knees bent and feet flat on the floor. She braces the abdominal wall, holding the lumbar spine in a neutral position, and slowly raises one foot 6 to 12 in off the ground with alternate legs. Common errors when performing this exercise include rocking the pelvis, abdominal protrusion, or an inability to maintain the neutral (midrange) lumbar curve. If this happens, discontinue the exercise for a rest period. Quality is stressed more than quantity. Progression: the exercise can progress to extending the legs alternately and lowering to the ground. Once the athlete can maintain stability with alternate leg lifts, she can add alternate, overhead arm raises for greater challenge. The arm raises should be performed slowly, while maintaining lower abdominal bracing.

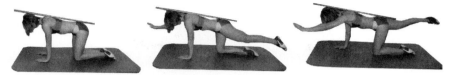

Fig. 5. Quadruped with alternate arm/leg raises. This exercise prepares the athlete for the proprioceptively more challenging and more dynamic exercises of the trunk. It specifically engages the multifidi—the deep transverse spine stabilizer and extensor of the lumbar spine. The athlete should position herself on all fours and brace the abdominal wall. While maintaining a midrange/neutral curve of the lumbar spine, the athlete should raise the right arm and the left leg (opposite upper and lower limbs) into a line with the trunk, while preventing any rocking of the pelvis or spine (excessive transverse or coronal plane motion). If it helps to maintain alignment, the athlete may use an object, such as a foam roller or wooden dowel, placed along the spine, for added tactile feedback. The leg should be raised only to the height at which the athlete can control any excessive motion of the lumbo-pelvic region. She then performs the exercise by raising the left arm with the right leg. Progression: a physioball underneath the trunk can provide significantly more proprioceptive challenge because of its unstable surface. The goal is to maintain lumbar stability while the opposite arm and leg are raised slowly.

rectus abdominis muscles—the muscles that are strengthened by traditional back and abdominal exercises and that assist with gross spinal movements.

Hodges and Richardson [6,7] showed that it is not simply that deep-layer abdominal muscles are recruited during stabilization of the spine, but it is how they are recruited that is important. The transverse abdominus, the innermost of the four abdominal muscles, has fibers that run horizontally (except for the most inferior fibers, which run in line with the internal oblique muscle). The transverse abdominus and the multifidi are considered "stabilizing muscles" (muscles that are modulated continually by the central nervous system and

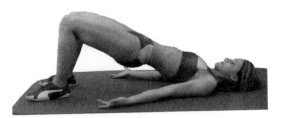

Fig. 6. Bridging. Bridging is a fundamental core-stability and gluteal-strengthening exercise. The athlete begins the exercise on her back, in a hook-lying position, with arms resting at her sides. She activates the abdominals and squeezes the gluteal cheeks before initiating the movement. The athlete lifts the pelvis and hips off the ground while maintaining neutral lumbar alignment. There should be no rotation of the pelvis. The hips should be aligned with the knees and shoulders in a straight line. The athlete should hold the position for 10 seconds and then slowly lower the pelvis to the floor. Progression: in the lifted-bridge position, while maintaining neutral lumbar and pelvic alignment, the athlete can lift one foot off the ground and extend the leg. By placing her arms across her chest, she can increase the challenge of stabilizing the lumbo-pelvic region.

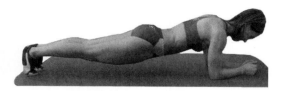

Fig. 7. Prone plank. This is a fundamental, static core stability exercise. The athlete supports herself with her forearms resting on the mat, elbows bent at 90°, and the toes resting on the mat. The athlete maintains the spine in a neutral position, recruits the gluteal muscles, and keeps the head level with the floor. She is instructed to breathe normally throughout the exercise, while maintaining the abdominal brace. We suggest holding the position for 20 seconds and working up to 1 minute for two or three repetitions. No compensatory motion should be seen, such as increased lumbar lordosis or sag. Progression: in this position, the athlete can add leg lifts for more difficulty. One leg can be lifted off the mat, held for 5 seconds, and then repeated on the opposite side. For more advanced progression, the legs (and for even greater challenge, the toes) can be balanced on a physioball.

provide feedback about joint position), whereas the global and larger torque-producing muscles control acceleration and deceleration. The investigators found that the cocontraction of the deeper-layer transverse abdominus and multifidi muscle groups occurs before any movement of the limbs. They noted that the transverse abdominus is active 30 milliseconds before movement of the shoulder and 110 milliseconds before leg movement; this neuromuscular stabilization may be delayed in individuals who have low back pain. It is believed that these muscles anticipate dynamic forces that may affect the lumbar spine and act to stabilize the spine before movement. In agreement with this, Hides and colleagues [8] documented that patients who sustained a low back injury had difficulty recruiting their transverse abdominus and multifidi muscles early enough to stabilize the spine before movement.

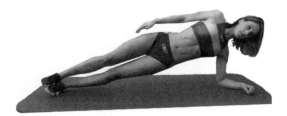

Fig. 8. Side plank. This is a fundamental, static core stability exercise that is designed to challenge the athlete's body against gravity in the coronal/frontal plane, and is an ideal exercise to train the quadratus lumborum. The athlete lies on her right side with the right arm extended in a straight line up from the shoulder, with the forearm resting on the mat. She raises the pelvis from the floor and holds it in a straight-line "plank" position. The hips should not be allowed to sag toward the floor. We suggest holding the position for 20 seconds, working up to 1-minute holds for two or three repetitions. If this position is too difficult, bend the lower legs and allow the support to come from the elbow and knee versus elbow and lower leg/foot. Progression: the top foot can be raised to challenge the core and gluteal musculature increasingly.

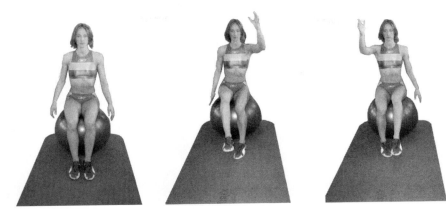

Fig. 9. Seated marching on a physioball. This exercise is more difficult because the athlete positions her body against gravity in a seated position on an unstable surface. The athlete begins by sitting upright on a physioball, with the lumbar spine in a neutral position (midrange). She places her feet hip-width apart. While bracing the abdominal muscles, she lifts one leg and foot off the ground. (The limb does not need to be lifted high, just enough to be off the ground—~2 inches to start.) The athlete should focus on controlling the weight shifting to the weight-bearing limb while maintaining lumbopelvic stability. Progression: once lumbo-pelvic stability can be maintained with alternate leg lifts, the athlete can add opposite arm lifts.

For a more detailed discussion on the theoretic basis for core strengthening, the reader is referred to a recent review article by Akuthota and Nadler [9].

## Muscle imbalances

Stability work should be started only after the athlete has achieved good mobility, because adequate muscle length and extensibility are crucial to proper joint function and efficiency. Also required is a proper relationship between the prime movers, synergists, and stabilizers. A prime mover is the muscle that provides most of the force during a desired body movement. Stabilizers and synergists are muscles that assist in the motion by means of control or neutralizing forces. Proper timing and coordinated effort of these muscles is paramount to the runner, and the functional exercises included here stress these relationships.

A thorough evaluation of the muscular system should include an assessment of the muscles for overactivity, shortening, weakness, inhibition, and quality of motion. This is accomplished best by using muscle-length tests, strength tests, and tests for the efficiency of basic movement patterns and neuromuscular control. A thorough postural observation and video-taping of the athlete's running gait will help in assessing and identifying any movement imbalances.

Muscles that are used frequently can shorten and become dominant in a motor pattern. If a muscle predominates in a motor pattern, its antagonist

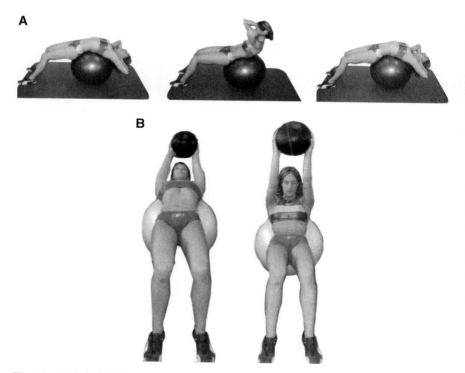

Fig. 10. (*A*) Spinal flexion on fit-ball. The athlete preactivates her abdominal brace in the starting position and maintains this as she rolls back into spinal extension. She slowly raises the body, focusing the rotation in the thoracic spine. Picture the head and neck as a rigid block on the thoracic spine to prevent flexing the cervical spine. The athlete concentrates on attempting to touch the bottom of her ribs to her pelvis anterior superior iliac spine. The hands can be placed over the ears to eliminate pulling on the neck. (*B*) Progression: a 5- to 10-pound medicine ball is held in front of the chest with the arms extended. By reaching up and diagonally, the oblique muscles can be emphasized.

may become inhibited and cause a muscle imbalance. An example of this is tightness in the iliopsoas muscle—the primary hip flexor that has its origins at the anterolateral aspect of the lumbar vertebral bodies and its transverse processes. When the iliopsoas muscle is tight or shortened, it is believed to inhibit the deep abdominals and the primary hip extensor—the gluteus maximus. Inhibition of the gluteus maximus muscles may result in inadequate stabilization of the lumbar spine, with increased anterior shear and extension forces on the lower lumbar vertebrae.

Muscles are divided into two types: postural and phasic (Box 1). Postural muscles are used for standing and walking. Phasic muscles are used for running; they propel the runner. Although 85% of the gait cycle is spent on one leg when walking [10], when running, there is a double-float phase during which both legs are off the ground—one at the beginning and one at

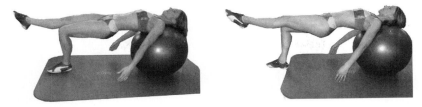

Fig. 11. Alternate leg bridge with shoulders on ball. The athlete starts this exercise by sitting on the physioball and walking forward with her feet on the ground, slowly leaning back until her back rests on the ball. This is called the bridge position. The head, neck, and shoulder blades should be supported on the ball. Knees should be bent at a 90° angle, with feet on the ground. While bracing the abdominal muscles, the athlete raises the foot and extends the leg off the ground. The weight is be shifted to one side, and the athlete should focus on maintaining stability of the lumbo-pelvic region. The athlete should strive for stability and balance, while holding this position for 10 seconds and alternating lower limbs. Progression: lift the arms up in the air or out to the sides.

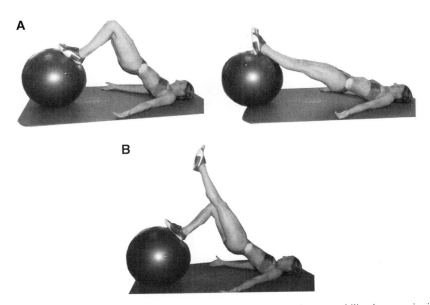

Fig. 12. (*A*) Leg curls on a physioball. The purpose of this dynamic core stabilization exercise is to recruit both actions of the hamstrings—hip extension and knee flexion—while maintaining dynamic stability of the lumbar spine. In a supine position on the floor, the athlete places both feet on the physioball. (Shoes should be removed to allow increased proprioception from the exteroceptors of the feet.) The athlete keeps her arms on the floor at the sides of the body for balance and raises the hips off the ground until the knees, hips, and shoulders create a straight line. She should focus on holding the spine in a neutral midrange position. In this position, the athlete pushes the ball forward with the feet while maintaining the bridge. The goal is to keep the pelvis elevated (hip extension) as both legs extend and flex at the knees. While the knees extend and flex from this elevated bridge position, the athlete focuses on maintaining lumbopelvic stability. (*B*) Progression: continue with single-leg hamstring curls in the same position.

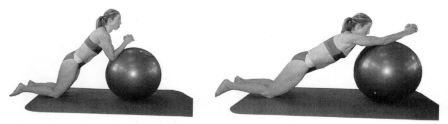

Fig. 13. Abdominal rollout. This is an excellent exercise to train the abdominals eccentrically. The athlete kneels behind the ball, with both hands on the ball. Keeping the abdominals braced and lower back in a neutral position, she rolls the ball away from her body a short distance until there is a straight line from the shoulder to hips. While maintaining alignment, she pulls the ball back towards them a short distance, then pushes it away a short distance. The movement should occur only at the shoulders, not the back. Progression: gradually straighten the body until up on the toes. There should be a straight line from the back of the head to the knees. Now move the ball away and back toward the body a short distance with the arms.

the end of swing phase. Running mechanics demand efficient firing patterns from the postural muscles, whereas phasic muscles do the work of propelling the runner forward. Because postural muscles are being activated constantly in the human body to fight the forces of gravity, they have a tendency to shorten and become tight. In runners, because of training and prolonged use, certain postural muscles are particularly likely to tighten, shorten, and become hypertonic. This occurs predominately in muscles that

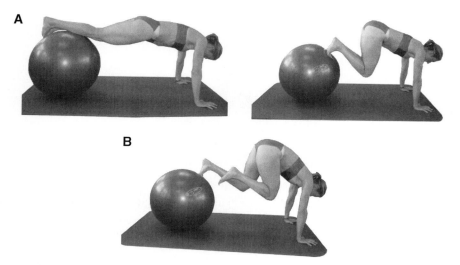

Fig. 14. (*A*) Squat ball thrust. Keeping the abdominals braced and lower back and shoulder blades in a neutral position, the athlete uses her abdominal contraction to move the ball forward and back. Keep the spine in neutral alignment throughout the movement. If the exercise is too challenging, start with the shins instead of the toes on the ball. (*B*) Progression: perform the exercise with only one foot on the ball.

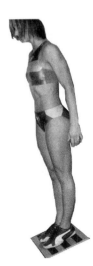

Fig. 15. Forward/backward rocking. In this exercise, the rocker board is used to challenge balance in a frontal plane of motion. Standing on the rocker board with both feet in perfect postural alignment, the athlete gently rocks forward and backward. (To maintain ideal posture, the athlete can create an imaginary line through the joints of the ankle, knee, hip, and shoulder. The ear should align in a straight line with these joints, with no excessive extension [swayback] of the lumbar spine or anterior pelvic rotation.) While rocking, there should be no excess body movement in the coronal or transverse planes. This exercise should be performed for several minutes. The goal is to align the spinal curves and lower extremities optimally. Progression: the athlete can progress to a slight flexed-knee position, with fast and slow movements to stimulate the righting reflexes and balance reactions. She also can progress the stepping motion to the three axes of motion.

cross more than one joint [11]. We commonly see this in the gastroc-soleus (predominantly the soleus), rectus femoris, iliopsoas, tensor fascia lata, hamstrings, adductors, quadratus lumborum, piriformis, and sartorius. Restricted extensibility of muscles also can lead to decreased circulation and ischemia, which contributes to overuse injury [12].

In comparison, phasic muscles (the more global muscles) typically may remain in an elongated state. It was shown that elongated muscles may lack force in shortened-range test positions [13]. Weak phasic muscles might allow excessive motion to occur at the joints upon which they act. In our experience, common phasic muscles that have a tendency to develop weakness or become inhibited in runners are the tibialis anterior; peronei; vastus medialis; long thigh adductors; and the gluteus maximus, medius, and minimus.

## Beginning a core strengthening program

The first step in a preventive or performance-enhancing program is to assess which muscles have become tight and shortened. These deficits can be

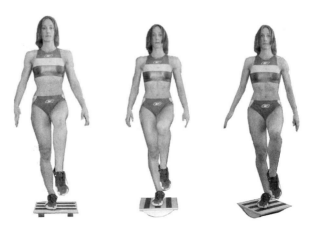

Fig. 16. Single-leg balance: three planes. This next exercise progresses the athlete to a single-leg stance. The rocker board is used in the three planes of motion. This exercise also can be performed with a balance board, which is more demanding because it incorporates all planes of motion simultaneously. The athlete takes one step forward while maintaining alignment and balance, controlling aberrant motion, and mimicking a forward running motion. The goal is to maintain lumbo-pelvic alignment. The athlete controls movement in the three planes of motions by placing her feet in various positions on the board. The athlete alternately steps forward and backward onto the rocker board. Progression: once the athlete achieves static stability and can remain stable while standing on the rocker board, she can add an accessory motion. The athlete can swing the arm and the nonweight-bearing opposite leg (as though mimicking running). No excessive motion in the pelvis or lumbar spine should occur during the swing phase.

addressed with stretching exercises and soft tissue mobilization techniques. Following this, the clinician should seek to activate inhibited, or strengthen any weak, muscle groups. The challenge for the clinician is to design an individualized program that addresses these imbalances.

Preliminary stretches for shortened, predominant muscles should include proprioceptive neuromuscular facilitation–type or contract-relax stretches that strive for isometric contraction, followed by end-range stretching. These are effective techniques for maintaining muscle length and joint mobility. Active Release Techniques [12], (a specialized method for soft tissue mobilization) when used in conjunction with stretching techniques, have shown great promise in restoring muscle length and soft tissue extensibility. Athletes also can do self-mobilization with the use of a foam roll. One example of this technique, which targets the iliotibial band, is shown in Fig. 1.

Middle-distance runners have unique and specific training programs that demand strength, power, and endurance. These runners place terrific demands for balance and precise functioning of structures all the way from the core to the feet. Specific exercises for the runner should progress from mobility to stability, reflexive motor patterning, acquiring the skills of fundamental movement patterns, and finally, progressive strengthening.

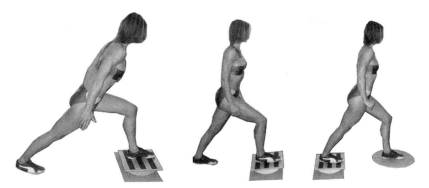

Fig. 17. Weight transfers with proper alignment. The preceding exercise progresses to "falling" onto an unstable surface. Pictured is a rocker board and "falling" onto a circular balance board. Again, emphasis is on spinal alignment from the head to the sacrum. The athlete steps forward quickly and catches himself from falling over with a quick forward movement of the leg onto the board.

These sequences may not be applicable to all athletes; therefore, the key is to analyze the individual in each exercise category and then to tailor an exercise regimen that will best suit that runner's needs. For example, it was shown that runners who are prone to iliotibial band syndrome often have weakness in their hip abductors that predisposes them to increased stress on the iliotibial band [14]. Thus, a preventative training program for runners who have this syndrome must target the hip abductors, particularly the posterior aspect of the gluteus medius that assists external rotation or in decelerating adduction of the hip. Other muscles that prove weak or inhibited on evaluation also should be strengthened on a case-by-case basis.

## The stages of core training

### Warm-up

Before beginning the basic core strengthening exercises, the athlete should warm-up the spine with the Cat-Camel motion (Fig. 2).

### Fundamental lumbo-pelvic stability

The purposes of the fundamental core stabilization exercises are to gain stability, but more importantly, to gain coordination and timing of the deep abdominal wall musculature. It is extremely important to do these basic exercises correctly because they are the foundation of all other core exercises and movement patterns. These basic exercises emphasize maintaining the lumbar spine in a neutral position (which is the midrange position between

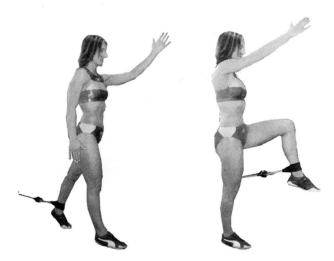

Fig. 18. Power runner with resistance. This exercise provides a functional movement pattern that is similar to running. The exercise seeks to increase stability of the lower abdominals while using a forward motion at the hip. The exercise is designed to develop sagittal plane control. While balancing on one leg, the athlete imitates a running motion. As the upper thigh is lifted forward in a running motion, the athlete concentrates on maintaining the abdominal brace and lumbo-pelvic stability while avoiding excessive anterior or posterior pelvic rotation. The athlete raises the opposite arm simultaneously into flexion, while maintaining postural alignment with an erect spine, and allowing only the extremities to move. Progression: once the athlete can maintain lumbar spine stability without effort, she can attach a pulley or resistive cord to the ankle to increase the challenge to the hip flexors.

lumbar extension and flexion.) This alignment allows for the natural curvature of the spine. All of these exercises are best done with light loads and high repetitions.

This first stage of core stability training begins with the athlete learning to stabilize the abdominal wall. Proper activation of these muscles is considered crucial in the first stages of a core stability program, before progressing to more dynamic and multiplanar activities. We recommend the abdominal bracing technique as described by McGill (Fig. 3) [4].

The exercise program should progress sequentially through the initial fundamental movements as detailed in Figs. 4 through 8. These fundamental exercises are to be performed three times a week to maximize results. The athlete begins with two sets of 15 repetitions and progresses to three sets of 15 to 20 repetitions to develop fully the requisite muscle endurance for higher level performance. Initially, these exercises are taught in a supine, hook-lying position or an all-fours quadruped position. The athlete can progress to more functional standing exercises as control is developed. Important concepts that are taught at this stage include not tilting the pelvis or flattening the spine. We also emphasize normal rhythmic breathing.

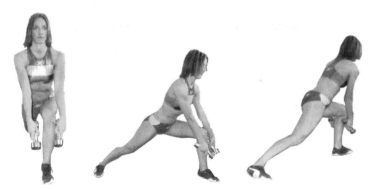

Fig. 19. Multidirectional lunges. The athlete begins this exercise with a forward lunge. Again, emphasis is on maintaining a neutral spine position and abdominal brace throughout the entire movement. The athlete steps forward, limiting knee flexion of the forward leg to 90°. The knee joint should be over the ankle joint and the patella should be aligned with the second toe. The lower part of the leg should be perpendicular to the ground. Progression: once strength and stability in the forward (sagittal) plane have been achieved, the athlete can begin stepping out at oblique angles, creating a narrower lunge or a wider lunge in the coronal or transverse planes.

## Advanced lumbo-pelvic stability

Once the athlete demonstrates good stability with all static core exercises, they can be replaced with more advanced exercises as detailed in Figs. 9 through 14. The use of the physioball requires the athlete to work on proprioception and higher level core stabilization. These exercises should be performed two to three times weekly to maximize results. Again, the athlete begins with one or two sets of 15 repetitions and progresses to three sets of 15 to 20 repetitions. Quality is more important than quantity. Make sure that the lumbar spine does not go into extension or the cervical/thoracic spine into flexion and maintain the spine in perfect alignment.

As the athlete progresses through a core exercise program, the emphasis always should be on correct postural alignment as athletes challenge themselves with a variety of movement patterns in the three planes of movement: sagittal, frontal, and transverse. Although runners move predominately in the sagittal plane, there still is body movement in the transverse and frontal planes that must be controlled adequately by the neuromuscular system. During midstance of the running gait cycle, the foot and ankle unlock to allow absorption of ground reaction forces. During this phase, the body is challenged most to control excessive or aberrant motion in the frontal and transverse planes. Functional exercises on one leg are used to best simulate the neuromuscular demands of running. The athlete is trained with increasingly challenging functional patterns, with continued emphasis on postural control and core stabilization. The ultimate goal of core stabilization is to train "movements" and "positions," rather than

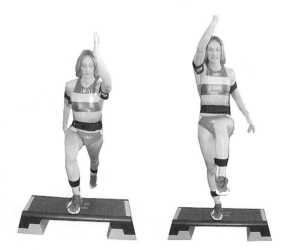

Fig. 20. Power runner with resistance and step-up. Continued progression: strength and stability with previous lunges must be achieved before starting this exercise. These exercises use a sports cord to resist shoulder and hip flexion while doing step-ups. The movement pattern is similar to the athlete's running gait. The opposite arm and leg are resisted simultaneously to increase strength and coordination of this movement pattern.

muscles. Exercises are most effective when they mirror the demands of the athlete's sport.

*Development of balance and motor control*

The following movements require reflexive control. The athlete can accomplish this control by using the numerous proprioceptors in the soles of the feet and the exteroceptors of the skin, and by activating the neck muscles; these are highly contributory to postural regulation. This sensory-motor stimulation is an attempt to provide the subcortex with a basis for movement that is progressively more challenging. It involves exercises that stimulate balance, coordination, precision, and skill acquisition.

The following exercises should be performed while standing (Figs. 15–17). We instruct the athlete to control the feet, pelvis, and head consciously, with the goal of making sure that the feet are aligned properly.

These exercises use a rocker board. A rocker board is a board with a hemisphere underneath that allows single-plane rocking. (The board was designed by Dr. Vladimer Janda to promote balance and stability of the spine, www.optp.com).

Common errors or abnormal compensations to look for when attempting these exercises include increased anterior pelvic tilt, increased lumbar lordosis, increasing internal rotation of the hip, excessive valgus at the knee, and hyperpronation at the foot. Therefore, when teaching these exercises, it

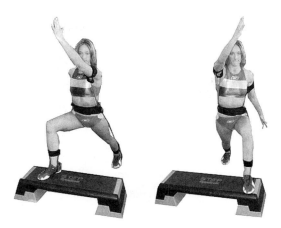

Fig. 21. Multidirectional resisted alternate arm/leg step-ups. Continued progression: once strength and stability are achieved in the frontal plane of motion the athlete can begin stepping up at 45°.

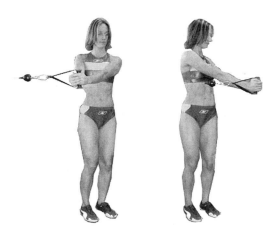

Fig. 22. Standing pulley or medicine ball rotation. This resistive, dynamic trunk pattern challenges the core with a rotational movement pattern while the athlete maintains stability in the hips and pelvis. It requires strict bracing of the abdominals and locking the rib cage and pelvis together to avoid unnecessary torsional stress on the spine. The athlete stands with feet about shoulder-width apart and knees slightly bent. She activates the abdominal brace before the movement. It is important to emphasize postural alignment, with the scapulae retracted and depressed. The athlete should maintain neutral spinal angles throughout the movement. Holding a straight-arm position (elbows extended) while grasping the pulley handle or medicine ball with both hands, the athlete rotates the trunk by activating the abdominal obliques and spinal rotators. She concentrates on keeping the arms extended in front of the chest. It is important that the pelvis remains stable in the movement. Resistance is perpendicular to the body. Progression: This exercise can be done in the same manner using increasing weight on the pulley or a 5- to 10-pound medicine ball.

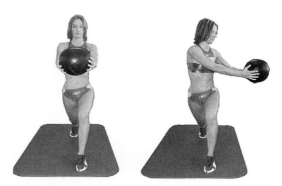

Fig. 23. Forward lunge with a medicine ball with trunk rotation. This exercise uses a resistive movement of the trunk with a lunge that demands a high level of lumbo-pelvic and lower extremity stability as the athlete moves the ball in a diagonal pattern across the body. Athletes need approximately 30 yards to complete this exercise. The athlete stands upright, holding onto a 5- to 10-pound medicine ball, with arms outstretched, perpendicular to the body. The athlete steps forward with the medicine ball in front of the chest with the arms extended. Once the lunge portion is completed, the athlete rotates the trunk by bringing the ball across the body toward the same side as the front leg and then returns the ball to midline as the next step is made. It is important that the knee joint on the stepping limb does not come forward past the vertical angle relative to the ankle joint. The second toe is aligned perpendicular with the patella. The purpose of this exercise is to challenge the trunk muscles with appropriate weight shift, balance, and control on one leg.

is imperative to instruct the athlete on proper spinal alignment. To aid in this, we recommend initiating the abdominal bracing technique before performing the stepping forward-and-backward motions of any of these exercises (which train correct weight transfer over the feet). Additionally, it is important to instruct the athlete on proper gait. The focus here should be on controlling the initial heel strike in a supinated position on the lateral edge of the foot, into pronation on the medial aspect of the foot, with flexion of the first metatarsal head and toes. Continuing proper gait instruction, we teach a falling-forward position into a lunge (with perfect control). The athlete then progresses to jumps on one or two legs, assuring that there is no increased lumbar lordosis or increased valgus moment at the knee. This stimulates vestibular and cerebellar activity, which, in turn, leads to automatic postural control—an important part of our training. (Readers will note the increased muscle activity of the ankles and muscles that control the lower extremity chain and spine.) The athlete can progress to standing on one leg, with alternating arm movements.

Various devices are useful to challenge balance progressively, moving the athlete from conscious to subconscious control of the muscles that are responsible for postural maintenance and gait. These devices include a balance board (a whole sphere underneath the board, which creates multiplanar instability) or a rocker board (a curved surface underneath the board, which allows single-plane motion). Dynamic foam rollers are an

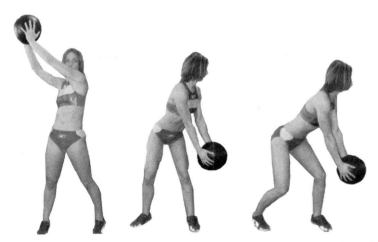

Fig. 24. Standing reverse wood chop with a medicine ball. This exercise is a resistive diagonal pattern of the trunk that demands a high level of lumbo-pelvic stability and combines upper- and lower-chain integration as the ball is moved in a diagonal pattern across the body. The athlete stands, holding onto a 5- to 10-pound medicine ball with both hands, with the feet approximately shoulder-width apart. While holding the arms in front of the body with elbows extended, the athlete moves the ball from a lower position at the hip, raising it across the body to the opposite shoulder, simulating a wood-chopping motion. The motion is then reversed by starting at the lower knee position and bringing the ball diagonally across the body, ending overhead toward the opposite shoulder. This exercise also can be performed with resistive cords or a pulley system that simulate the same motions. Progression: the athlete can progress to standing on one leg, using the opposite arm to complete the motion.

inexpensive alternative to the boards that also can be used to challenge balance, proprioception, and stability. These include half-rollers and full-sized rollers. Two other items that are invaluable to challenge balance and core stability and aid proprioceptive training in the standing position are the Bosu Balance Trainer and the Dyna Disk (these can be used interchange-ably). The Bosu has two functional surfaces that integrate dynamic balance with sports-specific or functional training: the domed surface is convex, the other side is flat and can be used for less challenge. The Dyna Disk is an air-filled plastic disc that can be inflated firmly. It has a smaller diameter than the Bosu and can be used like the Bosu Trainer because it creates an increased proprioceptive challenge to the athlete while standing on it. The Dyna Disk is unstable and does not have a base like the Bosu Trainer.

*Functional movement training*

Functional movements require acceleration, deceleration, and dynamic stabilization. Figs. 18 through 24 present an array of functional, diagonal exercises for the trunk and extremities that are essential for runners. Exercises should be safe, challenging, and stress multiplanar motions. These training exercises encourage functional strength, which depends on the

Table 1
Periodization of core training program

| Summer/Fall—base training (3×/wk, 3 sets of 15–20 repetitions for each exercise) | Winter—sport specific (2–3×/wk, 2–3 sets of 10–15 repetitions for each exercise) | Spring/Summer—competition (1–2×/wk, 2–3 sets of 8–12 repetitions for each exercise) |
|---|---|---|
| Restore mobility/address any muscle imbalances Fundamental core stability exercises Sensory motor stimulation | Advanced core stability exercises Functional movement training | Similar to sports specific training with addition of plyometric exercises |

neuromuscular system's ability to produce dynamic eccentric, concentric, and isometric contractions during movement patterns.

A functional exercise regimen that is specific to the demands of running includes single-leg drills, three-dimensional lunges, resistive diagonal patterns of the upper and lower extremities, drills that involve plyometrics, and triplanar movement sequences. Athletes can progress through the three planes of motion by performing similar exercises on balance boards, the Dyna Disk, or Bosu-type trainers, after static trunk and core stability have been mastered.

## Summary

This article is intended to provide an understanding of the importance of core musculature to runners and to offer exercises that will help them achieve desired mobility, stability, muscular balance, and neuromuscular control. Please see Table 1 for an example of how to incorporate these exercises into a periodized training program. It is highly recommended, however, that athletes consult a skilled practitioner to address individual needs and maximize results from a program of this nature.

## References

[1] Richardson C, Jull G, Hodges P, et al. Therapeutic exercise for spinal stabilization and low back pain: scientific basis and clinical approach. Edinburgh (Scotland): Churchill Livingstone; 1999.
[2] Lee D. An integrated model of "joint" function and its clinical application. Fourth Interdisciplinary World Congress on Low Back and Pelvic Pain. Montreal, Canada, p. 138.
[3] Nicholas JA, Strizak AM, Veras G. A study of thigh muscle weakness in different pathological states of the lower extremity. Am J Sports Med 1976;4:241–8.
[4] McGill S. Ultimate back fitness and performance. Waterloo: Wabuno Publishers; 2004.
[5] Comerford MJ, Mottram SL. Movement and stability dysfunction–contemporary developments. Man Ther 2001;6:15–26.
[6] Hodges PW, Richardson CA. Altered trunk muscle recruitment in people with low back pain with upper limb movement at different speeds. Arch Phys Med Rehabil 1999;80:1005–12.

[7] Hodges PW, Richardson CA. Inefficient muscular stabilization of the lumbar spine associated with low back pain. A motor control evaluation of transversus abdominis. Spine 1996;21:2640–50.

[8] Hides JA, Richardson CA, Jull GA. Multifidus muscle recovery is not automatic after resolution of acute, first-episode low back pain. Spine 1996;21:2763–9.

[9] Akuthota V, Nadler SF. Core strengthening. Arch Phys Med Rehabil 2004;85:S86–92.

[10] Janda V. On the concept of postural muscles and posture in man. Aust J Physiother 1983;29: 83–4.

[11] Kendall F, McCreary E, Provance P. Muscle testing & function. Baltimore: Williams and Wilkins; 1993.

[12] Schiottz-Christensen B, Mooney V, Azad S, et al. The role of active release manual therapy for upper extremity overuse syndromes-a preliminary report. J Occup Rehabil 1999;9: 201–11.

[13] Sahrmann S. Diagnosis and treatment of movement impairment syndromes. St. Louis: Mosby; 2000.

[14] Fredericson M, Cookingham CL, Chaudhari AM, et al. Hip abductor weakness in distance runners with iliotibial band syndrome. Clin J Sport Med 2000;10:169–75.

ELSEVIER
SAUNDERS

Phys Med Rehabil Clin N Am
16 (2005) 691–709

PHYSICAL MEDICINE
AND REHABILITATION
CLINICS OF
NORTH AMERICA

# Issues Unique to the Female Runner

## Heidi Prather, DO*, Deyvani Hunt, MD

*Physical Medicine and Rehabilitation, Department of Orthopaedic Surgery,
Washington University School of Medicine, 4829 Parkview Place, St. Louis, MO 64110, USA*

Although running offers extensive benefits, female runners have unique risks with respect to poor performance, repetitive stress, and acute injuries. The risks and types of injuries change as women age. Health care professionals must consider the anatomic, biomechanical, hormonal, and functional factors that are unique to women when caring for the injured female runner. Research regarding female athletes remains limited [1]. First, only two generations of elite female athletes have been studied; therefore, long-term outcomes over life spans have yet to be published. Second, compared with men, fewer women are involved in research, coaching, and sports medicine. Third, in the past, the variety of youth sports that was consistently available to girls has been limited. As more girls are involved in a greater variety of sports, more information will be established. This article outlines the anatomic, functional, hormonal, nutritional, and metabolic issues that are unique to female runners.

## Anatomic and biomechanical gender differences

Anatomic differences that are unique to the female athlete contribute to biomechanical differences that ultimately affect form and function. One fundamental difference between men and women is the pelvis. Typically, a female pelvis is wider than the male pelvis, and its shape is the basis for the lower extremity alignment gender differences. An example of these differences is a proximal mechanical difference, such as increased femoral anteversion found in women, combined with a hypoplastic vastus medialis obliquus muscle and genu valgum. This sets the stage for external tibial torsion, pes planus, excessive forefoot pronation, and heel valgus angulation found in the distal extremity. This alignment pattern is important for the female runner who relies on precise biomechanics for optimal performance.

---

* Corresponding author.
*E-mail address:* pratherh@wustl.edu (H. Prather).

1047-9651/05/$ - see front matter © 2005 Elsevier Inc. All rights reserved.
doi:10.1016/j.pmr.2005.03.002

Center of gravity differences between men and women are minimal and depend more on height and body type than gender [2]. Other distinctions that affect performance are attributed to hormonal differences. During puberty, girls gain fat mass and lean body mass because of increasing levels of estrogen, whereas boys gain lean body mass and lose body fat under the influence of androgens. Men also have higher hematocrit and hemoglobin levels than do women; these higher levels correlate to a higher oxygen-carrying capacity. Given all of these differences, studies have shown that women and men show the same physiologic response to training which results in similar relative gains in strength [3].

## Running throughout the life span

### The adolescent runner

As a female runner ages, different concerns that are unique to her emerge. Prepubertal female runners are similar to their male counterparts with regard to aerobic capacity, muscle mass, strength, and overall sports performance [4]. During puberty, however, female adolescent runners begin to experience changes in body composition and form. In this population, the female triad (eating disorders, menstrual dysfunction, and osteoporosis) becomes increasingly prevalent. Athletes attempt to maintain their pre-pubescent physiques by challenging physiologically induced body habitus changes with caloric restriction and radical calorie use techniques. A long-term consequence of the female triad, despite resolution of amenorrhea, is lifelong decreased bone mineral density (BMD). Osteopenia may progress to osteoporosis as the female runner ages.

### The pregnant runner

Pregnant runners must use caution when exercising. The American College of Obstetricians and Gynecologists published new guidelines for exercise during pregnancy in January 2002. Absolute and relative contra-indications to exercise are outlined in Box 1 [5]. One of the most important factors in the selection of a safe exercise program for pregnant runners is the prepregnancy fitness level. Pregnancy should not be a time to initiate a running program or increase a training schedule. Maintenance of activity, including running, is accepted and encouraged. Researchers continue to have mixed opinions on the correlation between specific types of exercise and its intensity, frequency, and duration on maternal fetal outcomes. Elite athletes have demonstrated the ability to train daily and rigorously until close to delivery without adverse consequence [3]. Box 2 summarizes the current recommendations for exercise during pregnancy [5]. The concerning consequences of intense exercise include the effect of elevated maternal

---

**Box 1. Relative and absolute contraindications to aerobic exercise during pregnancy**

*Relative*
Severe anemia
Cardiac arrhythmia
Chronic bronchitis
Poorly controlled diabetes
Morbid obesity
Extreme underweight
History of extremely sedentary lifestyle
Intrauterine growth restriction
Preeclampsia
Orthopedic limitations
Poorly controlled seizure disorder
Poorly controlled thyroid disease
Heavy smoker

*Absolute*
Hemodynamically significant heart disease
Restrictive lung disease
Multiple gestations at risk for premature labor
Persistent second or third trimester bleeding
Placenta previa after 26 weeks' gestation
Premature labor
Ruptured membranes
Pregnancy-induced hypertension

---

temperature on the fetus, the altered blood flow to the fetus in response to exercise and hydration status, and decreased fetal fat mass [6]. Patients who maintain an exercise program during pregnancy benefit from reduced weight gain, improved muscle tone, improved self-esteem, decreased incidence of varicosities, decreased incidence of low back pain, and improved sleep hygiene [7]. During pregnancy, runners may experience ligamentous laxity. Activity modification may be necessary.

Many of the physiologic changes that occur in pregnancy last 4 to 6 weeks post partum, but they can last longer in women who breastfeed. There are no studies to suggest that a rapid resumption of activity is detrimental; however, the detraining that occurs during pregnancy must be considered, and a gradual increase in activity is advised. Nursing mothers are recommended to breastfeed before activity to decrease the discomfort that is caused by engorged breasts and to limit the acidity of milk that is caused by elevated levels of lactic acid [6].

---

**Box 2. American College of Obstetricians and Gynecologists summary of recommendations for aerobic exercise during pregnancy**

Exercise should be at 65% to 85% of the maximum predicted heart rate

Exercise should occur at least 3 days a week for no more than 45 minutes at a time

Avoid the supine position

Women should monitor hydration status and body temperature (<38.7 °C)

Exercise should be stopped for extreme shortness of breath, dizziness, headache, chest pain, or contractions

Women should not exercise when fatigued and not exercise to exhaustion

Any exercise with the potential for abdominal trauma should be avoided

---

*The aging runner*

Female runners of advanced age also have special concerns. A common one is urinary stress incontinence. Involuntary loss of urine during exercise is underreported in female athletes [7]. This underreporting is believed to be related to the social implications and embarrassment regarding the problem. In one study, researchers reported that women who participate in exercise that requires long-term, repetitive motion and high-impact landings, jumping, and running report urinary incontinence more commonly [8]. Risk factors for this phenomenon include female gender, increasing age, increased parity, heavy physical activity, high-impact sports, hypoestrogenic amenorrhea, and obesity. Evaluation includes a pelvic floor examination to assess the integrity of the pelvic floor anatomy, muscle tone, muscle control, and muscle strength. Management includes pelvic floor therapeutic exercise, pharmacologic agents, or both [4].

Runners of advanced age who have nonspecific pain complaints should be evaluated for osteopenia, osteoporosis, stress fractures, pathologic fractures, and arthritic conditions. Hypoestrogenic women who have decreased bone mass are at increased risk for stress fractures. Sites at particular risk to runners include the metatarsals, the medial tibia, the femoral neck, and the pelvis. Insufficiency fractures may appear first as an insidious onset of low-level pain that progresses, and the pain may become chronic. Osteopenic aging runners who have buttock pain should have a sacral insufficiency fracture ruled out. Evaluation with plain films, bone scans, and CT will help to determine the diagnosis that underlies stress fractures. Referred pain may be the only presenting symptom. A common example is demonstrated by the runner who has refractory groin pain who eventually receives a diagnosis of a femoral neck insufficiency fracture.

## Clinical problems unique to the female runner

The causes for low back pain in the female runner are similar to those in the male runner and include muscle imbalance at the hip, pelvis, and spine; disc pain; radiculopathy; facet syndrome; sacroiliac joint dysfunction; and stress fracture at the pars or sacrum. When pregnant, women also are predisposed to back pain because of biomechanical changes, such as changes in the center of gravity, loss of abdominal stabilization, and increased ligamentous laxity. In particular, the sacroiliac joint is a common site of overload in a female runner, especially individuals who have ligamentous laxity. The relative instability in the sacroiliac joint can lead to posterior pelvic pain that is due to overload of intra-articular and periarticular pain sources. Runners who are at risk for low BMD also may encounter vertebral body fractures, pedicle stress fractures, compression fractures, and sacral insufficiency fractures.

Patellofemoral pain and dysfunction are more common in women [9]. Multiple factors contribute to this disparity, including ligamentous laxity, a deficient vastus medialis obliquus muscle, genu valgum, an increased Q angle, excessive pronation, and an external tibial torsion [3]. These factors create rotatory and laterally directed forces on the patella (Fig. 1) [1]. Along with malalignment issues, articular cartilage lesions, instability, and soft tissue factors contribute to the problem.

In a female runner, there are many causes of groin pain. Hip disease that produces groin pain includes, but is not limited to, arthritic conditions, mild dysplasia, labral disease, stress fractures, and avascular necrosis of the femoral head. Groin pain also can originate at the insertion of the adductor muscles. Long-standing adductor tendinitis can result in pubic symphysis and may progress to osteitis pubis.

Noncontact anterior cruciate ligament (ACL) injuries also are more common in women and have been linked to the same biomechanical differences between women and men [10]. Women are at risk for injury to their ACLs in positions of deceleration, landing, and cutting [11]. Runners who train or compete on uneven terrain may have the highest risk for these injuries.

Upper extremity issues are less common in female runners; however, potential scapulothoracic dysfunction, rib dysfunction, shoulder instability, and cervical spine problems should not be overlooked. The imbalance between the upper and lower quadrants that is created by a relatively weaker upper body with women can be a cause of lower extremity dysfunction and poor performance. To improve treatment, the health care provider should recognize the myofascial link that is created by the thoracolumbar fascia

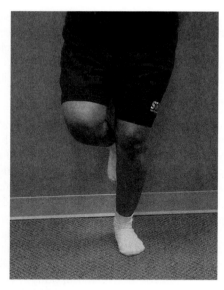

Fig. 1. Single leg squat demonstrates internal rotation at the hip, valgus stress at the knee, and pronation of the foot. The female pelvic girdle width enhances the valgus stress at the knee.

and the scapulothoracic region, thus integrating the upper limb to the pelvic stabilizers.

### Eating disorders

Eating disorders can occur in persons who participate in any sport; however, in those who participate in endurance sports, such as running, the risk of developing an eating disorder is substantial. Studies estimate the prevalence of eating disorders in elite female athletes to be as high as 60% [2]. Female runners are at greater risk for having an eating disorder than their age-matched nonathletic counterparts [3]. Eating disorders are psychiatric disorders that have physiologic consequences. Significant nutritional and medical complications occur, which range from amenorrhea and osteoporosis to bradycardia. In female runners whose disorders are untreated, the death rate is 12% to 18% [4].

The *Diagnostic and Statistical Manual of Mental Disorders, Fourth Edition* (DSM-IV), categorizes eating disorders into three distinct entities: anorexia nervosa, bulimia nervosa, and eating disorders not otherwise specified (NOS) [5]. The last category was added to help in the early identification of eating disorders, and thereby, improve patient care. Anorexia nervosa is defined by extreme weight loss or failure to gain weight with a body weight of less than 85% of that expected for height; a distorted body image; an overwhelming fear of obesity; and three consecutive months of amenorrhea in women after the establishment of menarche or failure of the onset of menses by age 16 years (Box 3) [6]. Bulimia nervosa is defined as recurrent episodes of binge eating at least twice a week for 3 months and recurrent inappropriate compensatory behavior in an attempt to prevent weight gain, such as vomiting, laxative abuse, or overexercising (Box 4) [6]. The category of eating disorders NOS includes individuals who meet all of the criteria for anorexia, except have regular menses, or are within the acceptable weight range for height. Also included are patients who meet all of the criteria for bulimia with the exception that they binge less than twice a week or for less than 3 months. Patients who have normal body weight who regularly display compensatory behaviors are at significant risk for having an eating disorder. These behaviors include eating small amounts of food, chewing and spitting out food without swallowing, or binge eating without purging. All of these are categorized as an eating disorder NOS.

A constellation of abnormal eating behaviors that are exemplified by: (1) calorie, protein, and fat restrictions and (2) pathogenic weight control measures including, but not limited to, self-induced vomiting, excessive exercising, laxatives, and diet pills puts an athlete at risk for adverse physiologic consequences. Athletes who are involved in sports that focus on physical form and physical performance are at increased risk for jeopardizing nutritional requirements in the quest for the "ideal" body image. Runners fall within this category; female runners, in particular, are at higher risk for eating disorders than their male counterparts [7].

---

**Box 3. Signs and symptoms of anorexia nervosa**

Primary or secondary amenorrhea
Delayed puberty
Hypothermia
Dry skin
Cold intolerance
Lanugo hair
Constipation
Bloating
Early satiety
Weakness, fatigue, or low energy
Nerve compression
Decreased bone density
Syncope
Orthostatic hypotension
Sinus bradycardia
Cardiac murmurs

---

**Box 4. Signs and symptoms of bulimia nervosa**

Amenorrhea or irregular periods
Mouth sores
Dental caries
Pharyngeal trauma
Heartburn, chest pain
Muscle cramps
Weakness
Bloody diarrhea
Easy bruising or bleeding
Syncope
Swollen parotid glands
Sinus bradycardia
Orthostatic hypotension

---

Psychologic factors are tied intimately to eating disorders. There is some concern that the psychologic profile of an athlete predisposes one to an eating disorder. A counter to this is that the demands of the sport itself set the stage. Most runners are highly motivated individuals who seek a high level of control and accomplishment. This psychologic profile, combined with the pressure to optimize performance and modify appearance, is a risk factor for eating disorders (Box 5) [8].

Medical complications of eating disorders affect all organ systems with the most consequential effects to the endocrine, skeletal, and cardiovascular systems (Box 6) [6,8]. Anorexia can cause hypothalamic amenorrhea and eventually lead to estrogen deficiency–induced osteoporosis [9]. This cascade of events can lead to an irreversible deficiency in BMD. Cardiovascular abnormalities, including arrhythmias, heart block, and orthostatic hypo-

---

**Box 5. Psychologic factors associated with eating disorders**

Low self-esteem
Poor coping skills
Perceived loss of control
Perfectionism
Obsessive compulsive traits
Depression
Anxiety
History of sexual/physical abuse

---

---

**Box 6. Medical complications associated with eating disorders**

*Cardiovascular*
Cardiac arrhythmias
Sudden cardiac death
Irreversible cardiac damage
Fluid and electrolyte imbalances
Nutritional deficiencies

*Endocrine*
Amenorrhea
Euthyroid sick syndrome
Osteopenia and osteoporosis

*Hematologic*
Leukopenia and pancytopenia
Iron deficiency anemia

*Gastrointestinal*
Dental erosions
Esophagitis
Slowed gastrointestinal motility
Ulcerations and bleeding
Bloating and constipation

*Cerebral*
Cortical atrophy
Altered cerebral metabolism

*Psychiatric*
Depression
Anxiety
Suicide

---

tension, may develop. Eating disorders have a strong psychologic basis, and it is not uncommon that concomitant psychologic disorders, such as depression and or anxiety, be present.

Practitioners should be familiar with the red flags that are related to eating disorders in the female runner (Box 7) [6]. While obtaining a thorough medical history and physically examining the patient, the provider also may find it helpful to investigate the patient's causes of stress; coping mechanisms; personality traits; and alcohol, tobacco, and drug use. Eating attitudes and behaviors may be difficult to ascertain; however, understanding the runners' behaviors and perceptions regarding nutrition is important for providing appropriate counseling and education. Menstrual history with

---

**Box 7. Eating disorder red flags**

Suspicion of an eating disorder by anyone
Isolation from friends
Frequent trips to the bathroom after meals
Recent change in dietary habits
Refusal to eat meals with family or friends
Change in bowel habits
Excessive food allergies and intolerances
Constant dieting
Use of dietary aids
Extra layering of clothes

---

abnormalities with primary or secondary amenorrhea is important to help qualify the extent of an eating disorder. Questionnaires, such as the modified Eating Attitudes Test, are a useful adjunct [1].

Physical examination should include a measure of height, weight, orthostatic blood pressure, and pulse. Estrogen status can be ascertained with Tanner staging in the peripubescent runner. It also may be prudent to rule out an endocrine disorder with examination of the follicular-stimulating hormone, the luteinizing hormone, thyrotropin, and serum prolactin levels. Endocrinology referrals often are appropriate.

Treatment protocols should focus on a multidisciplinary approach with support from physicians, physical therapists, coaches, athletic trainers, and mental health practitioners. The involvement of a psychologist or psychiatrist is essential because failure to address psychologic issues tends to undermine recovery. Education is a cornerstone for improvement. The return of menses usually correlates with the weight at which menses ceased. An increase in caloric intake to match energy expenditure is a necessary component for the reversal of amenorrhea. Calcium intake should be increased from 1200 mg/d to 1500 mg/d. Iron and protein intake also should be optimized. Training regimens should be evaluated. Most runners are reluctant to consider decreasing their level of training to a point where menses would return. In this group of women who also are hypoestrogenic, cyclical estrogen and progestin should be considered. Highlighting the use of estrogen for stress fracture prevention and bone health, and therefore, improved performance, instead of focusing on its benefits for the return of menses and weight gain may be necessary. If a patient experiences bradycardia (<50 beats per minute), orthostatic hypotension, severe dehydration, or electrolyte imbalance, hospitalization must be considered.

Prevention, early identification, and intervention are essential. A better prognosis for recovery of an eating disorder is associated with a shorter duration of symptoms, younger age, and less weight loss. A worse prognosis is associated with vomiting, an extreme degree of weight loss, and depression [6].

The investigation of eating disorders should focus on categorization by DSM-IV criteria, and identification of runners who have restrictive eating behaviors, poor nutritional habits, and routine use of excessive calorie-expending techniques. These patients easily slip through the practitioner's sieve without detection. Education regarding eating disorders should include peers, coaches, teachers, administrators, and parents. Again, patients who have eating disorders NOS are at risk for long-term cardiovascular, endocrine, skeletal, and psychiatric problems that can be avoided with early intervention and education.

Outside of the realm of eating disorders, iron deficiency anemia is another nutritional concern for female runners. High percentages (up to 80%) of female athletes are iron deficient [1,3]. Women can lose approximately 1 mg/d of iron through normal excretion; an additional 0.5 mg/d can be lost during menses. In the United States, a typical diet does not replace these losses. Over time, the iron stores become depleted, as evidenced by low serum ferritin levels. Low ferritin levels are associated with a significant decline in aerobic performance capacity [12]. Daily iron supplementation is recommended, especially for long-distance female runners.

## Menstrual dysfunction

Another component of the female athlete triad is menstrual dysfunction. Compared with menstrual dysfunction in nonathletes, menstrual dysfunction is two to three times more common in the athlete [13]. Menstrual dysfunction that occurs in girls can lead to low estrogen levels, which deter bone acquisition during the important adolescent years. Ultimately, acquired peak bone mass may be less than potential and contributes to the development of osteoporosis in later years [14]. In addition to the effects on BMD, runners who have menstrual dysfunction may have a higher incidence of stress fractures and a higher theoretic risk of infertility.

There are many types of menstrual irregularities. Amenorrhea is the absence of menses. Primary amenorrhea indicates that menses has not begun. Secondary amenorrhea indicates that menses occurred at one time and has ceased to continue. Menses must be absent for 3 or more months. Oligomenorrhea is menses that occurs irregularly. Oligomenorrheic women have six to nine cycles per year; the cycle is greater than 35 days or less than 3 months. Delayed menarche indicates that menses has begun after age 16 years, compared with the average ages of onset—12 to 13 years. It is common to observe that the onset of menses is delayed in elite athletes until age 15. Luteal phase dysfunction is defined as low progesterone levels with a normal cycle length. Anovulation is the absence of ovulation, but regular or irregular menstrual bleeding may occur [13]. All of these conditions are associated with intense training, low body weight, low body fat, poor nutrition, decreased calorie intake, an immature hypothalamic–pituitary–gonadal/adrenal axis, and elevated levels of circulating glucocorticosteroids from stress and exercise. Cortisol, androgens, and endorphins are secreted in response to stress. Their presence triggers a negative feedback on gonadotropin-releasing hormone. In addition, a hormone that is made by fat cells, leptin, is believed to be the link between body fat percentages, nutritional status, and menstrual dysfunctions. Leptin is believed to provide the feedback mechanism that affects the menstrual cycle through the hypothalamus [15–17]. As many as 60% of athletes experience irregular menses and anovulation as compared with approximately 5% of nonathletes [18]. The type of sports participation influences the percentage (eg, 20% of casual runners and 50% of elite runners and professional dancers report irregular menses) [4].

Amenorrhea and delayed menarche in adolescent girls can produce a hypoestrogenic state. This can decrease the rate of bone accumulation, as compared with bone resorption. Changes in the bone metabolism by hypoestrogenemia can be manifested as osteopenia, scoliosis, stress fractures, and lower peak bone mass acquisition [3].

Perceptions that menstrual cycles commonly are irregular, and therefore, are of no concern, can be harmful in the female runner. A discussion regarding the regularity of the menstrual cycle should be a focus of well visits with a health care provider. The young runner should be encouraged to report menstrual dysfunction to a confidante, such as a coach, parent, teacher, or peer. The significance of education to all of these individuals is important in detection and prevention. We recommend recording and tracking menstrual cycles in all female athletes [19].

"Athletic amenorrhea," or amenorrhea that is associated with athletes, is a diagnosis of exclusion. Medical causes for primary and secondary amenorrhea should be evaluated and are listed in Box 8. Other associated factors that are listed in Box 9 must be taken into account during the evaluation of the female runner. A normal menstrual cycle depends on an

---

**Box 8. Medical causes of primary and secondary amenorrhea**

Thyroid disease
Adrenal disease
Ovarian failure
Polycystic ovarian disease
Chromosomal abnormalities
Pituitary gland dysfunction
Prolactinoma
Malnutrition
Pregnancy

intact hypothalamic–pituitary–ovarian (HPO) axis and normal reproductive organ function. An energy imbalance theory states that when energy expenditure exceeds stored and consumed energy, a disruption in the function of the HPO axis occurs [12,20]. Intense exercise alone may not disrupt the HPO axis as long as enough calories are consumed to support the energy spent. An athlete who experiences amenorrhea or oligomenorrhea should undergo a progestin challenge test with 10 mg of medroxyprogesterone orally for 5 to 10 days. Induction of withdrawal bleeding should occur if sufficient levels of estrogen are present.

After menstrual disorders are diagnosed, treatment requires a comprehensive therapeutic approach. First, the athlete must be educated on the harm of energy imbalance that is established by running in excess of calories consumed. Reducing the intensity and quantity of the running regimen is recommended to balance better the energy in and out. Likewise, nutritional counseling is recommended to evaluate the current caloric intake and educate the runner on advisable changes, again with the goal of balancing energy intake and output. In many affected female runners, increasing body weight may be advisable. Another consideration is hormone replacement. If the runner has normal estrogen levels, progesterone can be used to initiate withdrawal bleeding and help to stimulate the menstrual cycle. If a hypoestrogenic state is found (estradiol level <50 pg/mL), oral contraceptives are recommended. Keep in mind that the American Academy of Pediatrics does not recommend hormone therapy within 3 years of menarche. It does recommend estrogen treatment in athletes who have experienced stress fractures [21]. Psychotherapy may be helpful in addressing body-image difficulties and other underlying factors that contribute to the dysfunction.

Educating athletes, coaches, parents, teachers, and administrators with regard to the deleterious affects of menstrual dysfunction is vital to the prevention of this problem. Discussions should dispel the idea that it is "normal" to have irregular menstrual cycles over a period of time. Attention also should be directed toward the evaluation of the athlete who has irregular menses. The irregularity may include anovulation, which also can

---

**Box 9. Multifactorial consideration for the etiology of menstrual dysfunction**

Body weight
Body composition
Nutrition
Training
Previous menstrual function
Psychosocial factors

produce a hypoestrogenic state that results in long-term effects. Screening for potential menstrual dysfunction should be incorporated into the preparticipation evaluation. The athlete should be made aware that menstrual dysfunction that is related solely to exercise is a diagnosis of exclusion; a full medical work-up should be completed before treatment recommendation to ensure that the treatment is appropriate. Early detection can reduce or reverse the negative effects on bone metabolism and prevent reduction in peak bone mass acquisition. This reduction has long-term health implications for women.

## Osteoporosis

Since the coining of the phrase "female athlete triad," more information regarding bone metabolism has become available. The incidence of osteopenia (1–2.5 SD less than adult mean BMD) and osteoporosis (2.5 SD less than young adult mean BMD) in the female athlete is unknown. Several studies showed osteopenia and osteoporosis in young female athletes who had menstrual dysfunction, eating disorders, or both [13]. It is now well-recognized that to reduce the number of female athletes who are at risk for osteoporosis, prevention must start during the adolescent years [22]. For some, prevention may need to begin before sports participation. Sixty percent of bone growth occurs during adolescence. Bone mass peaks at the end of this growth. Thus, bone mass is most important in preventing future bone loss later in adulthood [23].

Weight-bearing physical activity was shown to be helpful in modifying bone geometry during teen and adult years [24]. Mechanical loading in premature infants was shown to improve bone mass [25,26] and reduce bone loss [27]. These study results emphasize the important role that exercise plays in bone formation and mineralization during periods of rapid bone growth. Physically active middle-aged and elderly adults have significantly higher BMDs and bone mineral contents compared with controls [28]. Overall, physical activity is osteoprotective throughout a woman's life span.

Overdoing any good activity is not always beneficial. Too much exercise is no exception. Bone mass is dependent on a balance between resorption and deposition. Excessive exercise may affect bone turnover negatively through negative feedback on sex hormone secretion. An increase in osteoclast (a cell that promotes bone breakdown) activity is noted with low estrogen levels. Estrogen is important because it limits bone resorption, stimulates calcitonin, and promotes renal retention of calcium [29]. Another hormone, progesterone, was shown to reduce bone resorption and enhance bone formation. Testosterone, found in men and women, contributes to bone size.

An adequate nutritional status is crucial to bone health. Calcium and vitamins A and D have significant affects on bone metabolism. Calcium is essential for bone formation and improves BMD at all ages [30]. Whether absorbed in the skin by way of the sun or ingested orally through food, vitamin D preserves skeletal stores of calcium and is an essential component for bone metabolism. High doses of vitamin A stimulate osteoclast activity and results in bone breakdown. Additionally, these high doses of vitamin A can interfere with vitamin D [31]. An overall poor nutritional status may affect bone metabolism through the effects of leptin, which is mediated centrally [15].

Female runners are under pressure to maintain appropriate body fat and appearance. As a result, these athletes often place themselves on restrictive diets that may result in a poor nutritional status or an endocrine dysfunction that ultimately compromises bone health. A vigorous running or training schedule may lead to secondary amenorrhea. Amenorrhea that is related to strenuous activity is associated with low estrogen levels [14]. Furthermore, an eating disorder, such as anorexia, which is associated with amenorrhea, may result in plummeting estrogen levels that are nearly equal to those in women who have undergone menopause. Together, these deter acquisition of peak bone mass during puberty and excessive bone loss in later years.

Other factors can have a negative effect on the balance of bone metabolism for runners. Among some of the controllable ones are tobacco and excessive alcohol consumption. Certain medical conditions, such as renal disease and hyperparathyroidism, cause an increase in bone resorption. Medications, such as glucocorticosteroids and thiazide diuretics, also can compromise bone mineralization. All of these factors can put the runner at greater risk for stress fracture and should be considered during evaluation of a new or recurrent injury [32].

Evaluation for osteopenia and osteoporosis is assessed most commonly with dual energy absorptiometry scans. Scores are given through comparison of patients with age- and sex-matched controls. The World Health Organization diagnostic guidelines for postmenopausal women indicate a diagnosis of osteopenia with a $t$ score between $-1.0$ and $-2.5$ SD and osteoporosis with a $t$ score of less than $-2.5$ SD [33]. The BMD also can be calculated with CT, peripheral bone scanning, and quantitative ultrasound.

After osteopenia and osteoporosis are diagnosed, medical therapeutic intervention should be initiated to reduce fracture risk in girls and women who have one or more risk factors and have BMD $t$ scores that are less than $-1.5$ SD. Weight-bearing exercise and resistance training can improve bone mass; however, in the case of the female runner, a careful running history should be taken to assess for excessive training as a potential cause for a low BMD. Asking if the menstrual cycle is present and if it is irregular is important. Irregular cycles may indicate inconsistent ovulation, and thereby, an additional risk for low estrogen. Return of the menstrual cycle has been associated with an improved BMD. Regular menstrual cycles, with the aid of oral contraceptives, may have a role but have not been shown to improve BMD. Women who are at risk should consume 1500 mg of dietary calcium per day with 400 IU of vitamin D. A combination of calcium and estrogen supplementation in athletes who have amenorrhea and in those who have undergone menopause can increase bone mass 4% in 1 year [3,34]. Hormone replacement therapy (HRT) for the athlete at risk is controversial in women in whom menopause has not begun [35–37]. HRT should not be prescribed for skeletally immature young women because estrogens can cause physeal closure. An increasing number of alternative agents to HRT also seem to reduce fracture risk in postmenopausal women. These include bisphosphonates, calcitonin, selective estrogen receptor modulators (SERMs), and parathyroid hormone (Forteo, Eli Lilly, Indianapolis, Indiana). In addition to reducing fracture risks, these agents were shown to improve BMD. Bisphosphonates, calcitonin, estrogens, and SERMs (raloxifene) affect the bone remodeling cycle and are classified as antiresorptive medications. Bone mass increases over time because new bone formation occurs at a rate greater than resorption. None of these drugs have been studied in young women who have osteopenia or osteoporosis. Bisphosphonates are known to be teratogenic and remain absorbed in bone for months after cessation. For these reasons, bisphosphonates are not recommended in the young athlete. Parathyroid hormone is the only available agent that is approved for women who have undergone menopause and for men who are at high risk for fracture that promotes bone formation. This medication reduces fracture in the spine, hip, foot, ribs, and wrist of women who have undergone menopause and in the spine of men. At this time, its use in the young population has not been studied thoroughly.

In summary, the best management for osteopenia and osteoporosis in female athletes is prevention and early identification of risk factors. Eating disorders and menstrual dysfunction that are related to energy imbalance are most significant in the detection of bone disease. The runner may be obsessed with an increased training schedule, rigid dietary intake, or both. Education regarding these risks should include parents, coaches, administrators, health care professionals, and especially, peers. Any runner who is treated for concomitant stress fractures should be evaluated. Evaluation includes laboratory testing as necessary and assessment for training schedule, nutritional status, menstrual cycle history (be careful to note irregular cycles as well as cessation), and BMD. Treatment is multidisciplinary, including restoration of normal menstrual cycles, optimization of physical activity and nutrition, psychologic therapy, and medications when indicated.

## Cardiovascular risks

There is increasing evidence of an association of amenorrhea and osteoporosis with cardiovascular disease. Zeni Hoch et al [38] studied 20 female runners who had amenorrhea and oligomenorrhea. Compared with the women who had oligomenorrhea and the control groups, the group that had athletic amenorrhea showed a reduced endothelium-dependent dilation of the brachial artery. This finding suggests that the runner who has athletic amenorrhea may be predisposed to an accelerated development of cardiovascular disease. At the other end of the age spectrum, Jorgensen et al [39] studied 2543 men and 2726 postmenopausal women and compared the carotid ultrasounds and BMD. They found that a low bone mass was associated with an increased risk of echogenic calcified atherosclerotic plaques. These studies indicate that amenorrhea and low bone density that may begin during adolescence can have long-lasting cardiovascular effects.

## Summary

Care and treatment of female runners will improve as further knowledge regarding the unique factors that affect them becomes available. For care and treatment to be their most effective, current and recent information needs to be disseminated among health care providers, coaches, teachers, school administrators, and parents. In young athletes, peer support and education are the most important factors in the success of detection and treatment. Individuals who have the female athlete triad are at significant risk for stress fractures and other injuries. Early detection and multidisciplinary treatment should begin after fractures are detected to reduce or prevent long-term adverse sequelae to bone. In addition, correction of menstrual dysfunction can help to prevent later fertility problems. Addressing the unique biomechanics and core strength of female runners also is essential to rehabilitate athletes past symptom resolution. A thorough understanding of the unique issues for female runners is essential for the prevention of injuries and plays an important role in the promotion of female participation in recreational and competitive running.

## References

[1] Ireland ML, Ott SM. Special concerns of the female athlete. Clin Sports Med 2004;23: 281–98.

[2] Atwater A. Biomechanics and the female athlete. In: Puhl J, Brown C, Voy R, editors. Sports science perspectives for women. Champaign (IL): Human Kinetics Books; 1988. p. 1–12.

[3] Holschen J. The female athlete. South Med J 2004;9:852–8.

[4] Greydanus D, Patel D. The female athlete. Before and beyond puberty. Pediatr Clin North Am 2002;49:558–80.

[5] ACOG Committee Obstetric Practice. ACOG Committee opinion. Number 267, January 2002: exercise during pregnancy and the postpartum period. Obstet Gynecol 2002;99:171–3.

[6] Artal R, O'Toole M. Guidelines of the American College of Obstetricians and Gynecologists for exercise during pregnancy and the postpartum period. Br J Sports Med 2003;37:6–12.

[7] Nattiv A, Arendt E, Hecht S. The female athlete. In: Garrett W, Kirkendall D, Squire D, editors. Principles and practice of primary care sports medicine. Philadelphia: Lippincott Williams and Wilkins; 2001. p. 93–113.

[8] Nygaard I, DeLancey J, Arnsdorf L, et al. Exercise and incontinence. Obstet Gynecol 1990; 75:848–51.

[9] Baker M, Juhn M. Patellofemoral pain syndrome in the female athlete. Clin Sports Med 2000;19:315–29.

[10] Griffin L, Agel J, Albohm MJ, et al. Noncontact anterior cruciate ligament injuries: risk factors and prevention strategies. J Am Acad Orthop Surg 2000;8:141–50.

[11] Chappell J, Yu B, Kirkendall D, et al. A comparison of knee kinetics between male and female recreational athletes in stop-jump tasks. Am J Sports Med 2002;30:261–7.

[12] Friedmann B, Weller E, Mairbaurl H, et al. Effects of iron repletion on blood volume and performance capacity in young athletes. Med Sci Sports Exerc 2001;33:741–6.

[13] American Academy of Family Physicians. American Academy of Orthopedic Surgeons, American College of Sports Medicine, American Medical Society for Sports Medicine, American Orthopedic Society for Sports Medicine, American Osteopathic Academy of Sports Medicine. Female athlete issues for the team physician: a consensus statement. Med Sci Sports Exerc 2003;35:1785–93.

[14] Eliakim A, Beyth Y. Exercise training, menstrual irregularities and bone development in children and adolescents. J Pediatr Adolesc Gynecol 2003;16:201–6.

[15] Ireland ML, Nattiv A, editors. The female athlete. Philadelphia: Saunders; 2002.

[16] Laughlin GA, Yen SSC. Hypoleptinemia in women athletes: absence of diurnal rhythm with amenorrhea. J Clin Endocrinal Metab 1997;82:318–21.

[17] Thong FS, McLean C, Graham TE. Plasma leptin in female athletes: relationship with body fat, reproductive, nutritional and endocrine factors. J Appl Physiol 2000;88:2037–44.

[18] Otis CL. Exercise-associated amenorrhea. Clin Sports Med 1992;11:351–62.

[19] Snow-Harter CM. Bone health and prevention of osteoporosis in active and athletic women. Clin Sports Med 1994;13:389–404.

[20] De Souza MJ, Williams NI. Physiological aspects and clinical sequelae of energy deficiency and hypoestrogenism in exercising women. Hum Reprod Update 2004;10:433–48.

[21] American Academy of Pediatrics. Committee on Sports Medicine: amenorrhea in adolescent athletes. Pediatrics 1989;84:394–5.

[22] Nattiv A. Stress fractures and bone health in track and field athletes. J Sci Med Sport 2000; 3:268–79.

[23] Janz K. Physical activity and bone development during childhood and adolescence: implications for the prevention of osteoporosis. Minerva Pediatr 2002;54:93–104.

[24] Pettersson U, Nordstrom P, Alfredson H, et al. Effect of high impact activity on bone mass and size in adolescent females: a comparative study between two different types of sports. Calcif Tissue Int 2000;67:207–14.

[25] Moyer-Mileur L, Luetkemeier M, Boomer L, et al. Effect of physical activity on bone mineralization in premature infants. J Pediatr 1995;127:620–5.

[26] Moyer-Mileur L, Brunstetter V, McNaught TP, et al. Daily physical activity program increases bone mineralization and growth in preterm very low birth weight infants. Pediatrics 2000;106:1088–92.

[27] Litmanovitz I, Dolfin T, Friedland O, et al. Early physical activity intervention prevents decrease of bone strength in very low birth weight infants. Pediatrics 2003;112(1 Pt 1):15–9.

[28] Suominen H. Bone mineral density and long term exercise. An overview of cross-sectional athlete studies. Sports Med 1993;16:316–30.

[29] Khan K, McKay H, Kannus P, et al. Physical activity and bone health. Champaign (IL): Human Kinetics; 2001.

[30] Prince RL. Diet and the prevention of osteoporotic fracture. N Engl J Med 1997;337:701–2.

[31] Peer KS. Bone health in athletes. Factors and future considerations. Orthop Nurs 2004;23: 174–81.

[32] Gibson J. Osteoporosis. In: Drinkwater B, editor. Women in sport. London: Blackwell; 2000. p. 391–406.

[33] Assessment of fracture risk and its application to screening for postmenopausal osteoporosis. Report of a WHO Study Group. World Health Organ Tech Rep Ser 1994; 843:1–129.

[34] Agostini R. editor. The athletic woman. Clin Sports Med 1994;13(2):61–9.
[35] National Osteoporosis Foundation: The physician's guide to prevention and treatment of osteoporosis. Available at http://www.nof.org/physguide/index.htm. Accessed November 15, 2004.
[36] NIH Consensus Development Panel on Osteoporosis Prevention, Diagnosis, and Therapy. Osteoporosis prevention, diagnosis, and therapy. JAMA 2001;285:785–95.
[37] Rossouw JE, Anderson GL, Prentice RL, et al. Risks and benefits of estrogen plus progestin in healthy postmenopausal women: principal results from the Women's Health Initiative randomized controlled trial. JAMA 2002;288:321–33.
[38] Zeni Hoch A, Dempsey RL, Carrera GF, et al. Is there an association between athletic amenorrhea and endothelial cell dysfunction? Med Sci Sports Exerc 2003;35:377–83.
[39] Jorgensen L, Joakimsen O, Rosvold Berntsen GK, et al. Low bone mineral density is related to echogenic carotid artery plaques: a population-based study. Am J Epidemiol 2004;160: 549–56.

ELSEVIER
SAUNDERS

Phys Med Rehabil Clin N Am
16 (2005) 711–747

PHYSICAL MEDICINE
AND REHABILITATION
CLINICS OF
NORTH AMERICA

# Evidence-Based Treatment of Hip and Pelvic Injuries in Runners

Michael C. Geraci Jr, MD, PT[a,b,c,*],
Walter Brown, MSPT, OCS[a]

[a]Buffalo Spine and Sports Institute, 100 College Parkway, Suite 100,
Williamsville, NY 14221, USA
[b]Department of Physical Medicine and Rehabilitation,
State University of New York at Buffalo, Buffalo, NY 14260, USA
[c]College of Osteopathic Medicine, Michigan State University, East Lansing, MI 48824, USA

All too often, the runner who presents with pain or dysfunction in the hip or pelvis is approached from a one-joint or soft tissue injury concept. Because most injuries in this region are related to overuse, and, in particular, microtraumatic overload injury, a functional biomechanical approach is necessary to identify significant muscle imbalances and joint dysfunctions. A thorough understanding of the relationship between the lumbar spine, pelvis, hip, and thigh, and their relationship to the functional kinetic chain (including areas well-above and below the hip and pelvis) is key to evaluation and treatment. Using this concept, the long-term results of our treatment and the prevention of reinjury in runners will be more successful.

Approximately 5% to 21% of all athletic injuries involve the hip and pelvis [1,2]. In one study, overuse accounted for 82.4% of the injuries to the hip and pelvis that presented to a general sports medicine clinic [1]. Another investigator cited that 25% to 70% of runners sustain overuse injuries during any 1-year period [3]. Regardless of the level of athletic competition—recreational, high school, college, or professional—overuse injuries to the hip and pelvis region are equally common.

The exact causes of overuse running injuries have yet to be determined. The etiology of these injuries seems to be multifactorial and diverse in nature [4–6]. As an example, one of the most common and overlooked injuries in runners is gluteus medius tendinosis. Often, this is associated with a rigid supinated foot and a tight gastroc-soleus that does not allow

---

* Corresponding author. Buffalo Spine and Sports Institute, 100 College Parkway, Suite 100, Williamsville, NY 14221.
   E-mail address: mgeraci@pol.net (M.C. Geraci Jr).

calcaneal eversion and subsequent subtalar joint pronation. The functional kinetic chain is inhibited in internal rotation at the tibia and femur, which results in reduced stimuli to the gluteus medius muscle. The runner makes compensations in his running pattern until it is no longer possible, and finally, seeks medical attention. This emphasizes the importance of the functional kinetic chain, particularly the foot and ankle, to hip function [7].

This article does not focus on isolated stretching at the hip and pelvis as a means of prevention of injuries in runners. In fact, the focus is on exercises that simultaneously stretch and strengthen, to provide three-dimensional strengthening and flexibility. Isolated syndromes also are not addressed because the authors do not believe that these describe adequately the complex functional kinetic chain relationships that lead to pain in the hip and pelvis. Instead, the focus is on identifying the functional biomechanical deficits that lead to running-related hip and pelvis pain.

## Functional anatomy and biomechanics

Although the functional anatomy and biomechanics of running have been discussed previously, a brief review of the hip and pelvis area is provided here. The important link between the pelvis, trunk, and lower extremities is emphasized. The bone architecture of the hip joint shows primary compression and tension trabeculae of the femur that carry on through the pelvis, iliac crest, and lumbar spine. This trabecular pattern allows the hip to handle peak focal pressures of approximately 3000 pounds per square inch, which occur from sitting to standing. The multiaxial ball and socket joint of the hip has three degrees of freedom, whereas stability is provided through the acetabular triangular fibrocartilage which adds more congruency to the articular surfaces. The attachments of muscles, fascia, and ligaments in this region help one to appreciate the relationship between the lumbar spine, pelvis, hip, and thigh. The intrinsic ligaments of the hip (the iliofemoral, ischiofemoral, and pubofemoral) reinforce its strong joint capsule. The femoral, obturator, and sciatic nerves contribute to the vast innervation of the hip region.

The biomechanics of the neck-shaft angle of 120° to 130° along with an average of 14° of anteversion allow for angular movements of the thigh to be converted to rotatory (transverse plane) hip motion. At 30° of flexion and abduction, the hip joint is considered to be in the resting position. Hip joint pathology causes a capsular pattern of loss with hip flexion and internal rotation lost more than hip abduction. In general, the capsular pattern of any joint is a loss of motion in a characteristic pattern that indicates a tight joint capsule or intra-articular pathology, such as osteoarthritis. In the hip, full extension with internal rotation and abduction of the hip joint is considered the close-packed position. The close-packed position in any joint represents a position where the least amount of motion occurs as a result of ligamentous, capsular, and muscle tightness.

The pelvis is divided into three joints: the two sacroiliac joints, and symphysis pubis. The sacroiliac joint is an atypical synovial joint, and, in most cases, is patent throughout life [8]. Fusion can occur by synostosis or fibrosis. The ridges and depressions of this joint clearly are visible at the macroscopic level and are less pronounced in women [9]. The ligamentous relationship is a reminder of the connection between the lumbar spine, pelvis, hip, and thigh regions. The iliolumbar ligaments link L5 vertebral segment and, at times, L4, to the pelvis. The weaker anterior sacroiliac joint ligaments are thinner than their posterior counterparts and form an inferior sling under the sacroiliac joints. The multilevel short and stronger posterior ligaments and the long sacrotuberous and sacrospinous ligaments provide stability across the sacroiliac joint. The innervation of the sacroiliac joint is considerably vast (ie, from L2 through S2 levels); however, the main nerve supply, particularly of the posterior aspect of the joint, is received from L5, S1, and S2 dorsal rami.

Some of the important muscular relationships include the abdominals and adductors. Balance between these two muscle groups is essential, because the adductors attach from below to the pubic rami and the abdominals from above. Muscle imbalances—in which certain muscle groups become tight and others become inhibited and weak—occur frequently [10]. The tendency for the adductors to become tight and the lower abdominals to become inhibited and weak is an excellent example of a common muscle imbalance about the hip girdle.

One should consider that the pelvis and the sacroiliac joints serve as a functional link through which loads are transmitted from the lower extremities to the spine, and vice versa. The sacrotuberous ligaments are an important link in the kinetic chain between the lower extremities, pelvis, and lumbar spine [8,11–13]. The gluteus maximus attached to this ligament in all specimens studied and, in some cases, so did the piriformis and long head of the biceps [8]. In the anterior pelvis, the symphysis pubis has a superior to inferior translatory movement that may become dysfunctional secondary to imbalances of the adductors and lower abdominals. Anatomic and biomechanical research studies document sacroiliac joint motion throughout life [14,15]. The sacroiliac motion averages 2.5°, with a range of 0.8° to 3.9°. Translation averages 0.7 mm, with a range from 0.1 mm to 1.6 mm. An increase in sacroiliac joint motion by 25% is seen under relaxin influence, such as with pregnancy. Dysfunctions of the pelvis often are associated with hip, buttock, and groin pain syndromes.

Causes of overuse injuries in runners can be divided into three general categories [3]. The first category—training errors—include improper running shoes, excessive running distance or intensity, and a rapid increase in weekly running distances or intensity. The authors also include inadequate lower extremity weight training, especially in runners who are older than 30 years of age. Runners who continue to run regularly will lose approximately 30% strength (0.7% per year) if they do not properly train with weights. All too often, runners make the mistake of believing that they are strengthening their lower extremities with running, and therefore, only engage in upper body weight training. This is a grave mistake that has led many runners to frequent injuries. It is the authors' contention that the focus of a runner's cross-training routine should consist of strengthening and dynamic stretching, rather than a traditional prerun static stretching regimen.. Runners who stretch regularly before running have a higher injury rate than those who do not stretch [16].

Anatomic considerations are the second category. These include a high longitudinal arch (pes cavus), dysfunction in range of motion of ankle dorsiflexion or plantar flexion, tibia varum, rear foot varus, and leg length discrepancies. A flat foot (pes planus) also may be a risk factor.

The final category of biomechanical considerations includes kinetic variables, in particular, magnitude of impact forces, rate of impact loading, and active (push-off) forces. Rear foot kinematic variables include the magnitude and rate of foot pronation (calcaneal eversion). Although pronation is a needed physiologic factor to dampen ground reaction forces, uncontrolled pronation may be a factor that induces running injuries. Hreljac [3] looked at anatomic and biomechanical factors that are associated with running injury. These included height, weight, longitudinal arch height, footprint index, hamstring and ankle flexibility, and other biomechanical characteristics. The two most important characteristics in the group of runners that ran for 10 years injury-free were a decreased maximal vertical loading rate and a moderate rate of rear foot pronation. This is a clear indication that functional kinetic changes at the foot and ankle impact the injury rates on the whole functional kinetic chain in runners.

**Functional evaluation**

Efficient running requires that momentum of the body is maintained in a sagittal direction with minimal vertical displacement of the center of mass and with minimal deflection of the body into the frontal and transverse planes. This requires a sufficient level of spinal stability to offset the powerful loads that are placed on the spine by the propulsive force that is generated by the hip and pelvic muscles [17]. Function of these core muscles is enhanced by the coordination of the joints and muscles of the lower extremity and pelvis and by concomitant linked motions that occur in the shoulder girdle. This biomechanical linkage of the leg, core, and upper quarter has been described in terms of pronation (eccentric loading) and supination (concentric contraction) by Gray [18]. Eccentric loading is crucial for activating peripheral afferents that modify the centrally generated pattern of locomotion. Eccentric loading further provides the potential energy that is required to produce efficient concentric muscle contraction [19]. The motions of supination and pronation occur in three planes at each joint (see the article elsewhere in this issue on the biomechanics of running).

Gray and Tiberio also described a second phase of pronation in stance when the foot is supinated and behind the body that eccentrically loads the muscles of the hip and calf to facilitate the swing phase of gait.

With jogging, the ability to control pronation is crucial because the hip joint incurs contact forces of up to five times body weight [20]. The muscles and joints that make up the hip and pelvis play a key role in attenuating and transmitting this tremendous force during running. To that end, the body is designed with a massive bony pelvis and large powerful hip girdle musculature to attenuate force loads. Because of their short lever arms, hip muscles must generate greater forces to maintain hip stability during impact and throughout stance. This predisposes this region to soft tissue injury and potentially injurious intra-articular loads [21].

An orthopedic examination is useful for identifying the tissues that are affected by the potential mechanical overload of running. A regional orthopedic examination is unable to identify the mechanical limitations in the kinetic chain that may have predisposed the hip to injury, however [22]. Furthermore, the regional examination is unable to predict who is at risk for a running injury before participation, nor is it able to identify specific modifications that may help to rehabilitate or enhance a runner's performance [23]. To evaluate and treat the runner, or any athlete, it is necessary to apply loads in a way that parallel the specific demands of the activity. Ideally, the examiner should be able to identify by observation and, in some cases, by measurement, the specific joints and planes of motion that place the hip in jeopardy when running. Testing should establish bio-mechanical deficits, such as abnormal muscle function or poor mechanics of the hip. Seven functional tests that are used by the authors' clinicians who evaluate hip function as part of a linked kinetic chain are described.

## Functional examination

1. Observation:

   a. Static alignment of the lower extremity: Static alignment is suggestive but does not reveal how the pelvis, hip, knee, ankle, and foot interact in response to body weight and ground reaction force [24]. Williams and coworkers [25] noted that stiff-arched runners demonstrated increased loading rates which may predispose them to injury.

   b. Running: Whenever practical, the clinician should watch the patient run. Compensatory strategies that are a source of overload might be seen at this time. Observation should be made regarding length of stride. Impact forces and vertical displacement increase with stride length [26]. A shortened stride may be related to a proximal or distal sagittal blockade at any of the joints of the lower extremity. The amount of trunk motion in all three planes relative to the pelvis is a key observation. Insufficient or excessive motion in a specific plane about the trunk may suggest difficulty or inability to load the abdominals eccentrically to stabilize the pelvis.

2. Unilateral squat (Fig. 1): The pronation phase of a single leg squat mimics, to some extent, the key events of the loading phase of running and walking. Special attention is paid to how the patient controls eccentric loading of the muscles of the hip and pelvis. Important events to observe by plane of motion:

   a. Sagittal plane (SP): Excessive forward bending of the trunk relative to the amount of knee flexion is suggestive of quadriceps and gluteus maximus weakness or an overreliance on the hamstrings to decelerate anterior tilting of the pelvis and forward momentum of the trunk. This may result in a forward sway of the trunk in the initial stages of propulsion.
   b. Frontal plane (FP): A Trendelenburg sign (frontal plane lurch) may be elicited with a single leg squat. This usually indicates gluteus medius and minimus weakness.
   c. Transverse plane (TP): Rotation to the same side leg, to stabilize the hip over the femur, suggests weakness in the gluteus maximus in this plane of motion.
   d. Special attention should be given to excursion (range of motion) and control of subtalar joint pronation. The rate of subtalar motion should be proportional to the rate of internal rotation/abduction at

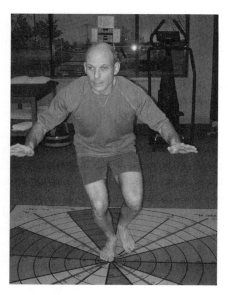

Fig. 1. Single leg squat. Controlled knee abduction and hip adduction should be noted in the frontal plane.

the tibia and femur. An immediate flattening of the longitudinal arch of the foot may be related to compromised control of pronation at the hip. Pronation that occurs too rapidly often is noted in the FP at the knee by excessive knee valgus as a result of poorly controlled femoral abduction. This is correlated with a weakened gluteus medius. It was noted that female recreational runners exhibited greater TP and FP motion at the hip and knee. The ability to control this excursion range may play a key role in avoiding overload of the lower extremities, and ultimately, injury [27].

3. Core mobility testing: The relationship of mobility of the lumbopelvic region and distal joints is examined in each plane of motion.

  a. Sagittal core (Fig. 2): The test is performed in a bilateral stance posture. The clinician demonstrates the test with minimal verbal coaching. Restriction of posterior to anterior translation during extension of the spine and extremities suggests tightness in the anterior hip capsule or psoas. Hyperextension of the lumbar spine and knee flexion are common compensatory patterns to achieve anterior translation of the trunk. During the flexion phase of this examination, an early heel rise is noted if there is inadequate ankle dorsiflexion, which often is associated with gastrocnemius tightness. Excessive hip flexion often is seen as a compensatory motion for restricted ankle dorsiflexion.

  b. Frontal core (Fig. 3): The starting position and instruction procedure is the same as with sagittal core testing. The primary observation is the ability to translate the pelvis in the frontal plane during truncal side-bending. Lateral translation of the pelvis to one side requires ipsilateral adduction and contralateral abduction of the hips. A restriction in abduction reflects tightness in the inferior or medial hip joint capsule, hip adductors, or medial hamstrings.

  c. Transverse core (Fig. 4): This test provides a wealth of information for functional diagnosis and treatment. It is performed in symmetric stance posture with feet shoulder width apart. The following points are kept in mind when observing the runner:

    (1) When compared with running and walking, the joint mechanics on the leg to the side of pelvic rotation are similar to those of the late stance phase of the propelling leg. The mechanics on the leg opposite the direction of pelvic rotation is similar to the loading portion of early stance. With supination, the pelvis, tibia, and femur are rotating externally (from top down), which results in subtalar joint inversion and locking of the foot. With supination, the pelvis goes through greater excursion (range) than the femur and tibia. This rotation of the pelvis relative to the femur maintains an ideal length tension for the gluteals, which are active in the later stages of propulsion [28].

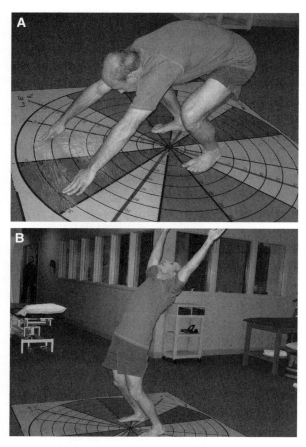

Fig. 2. Core testing in the sagittal plane. (*A*) Flexion phase. Tightness in the posterior hip capsule may restrict anterior to posterior pelvic translation. (*B*) Extension phase. Tightness in the anterior hip capsule may restrict posterior to anterior translation of the pelvis.

(2) In the transverse core test, the subtalar joint on the side of pelvic rotation should be able to invert the calcaneus and lock up the midtarsal joint, as it does in the last phases of stance, without a notable change in the anterior to posterior orientation of the foot. Attention should be paid to the feet and midtarsal joints to see if they remain stable or twist or roll to the side of rotation. Excessive lateral movement of the foot in this test may be associated with tightness of any of the muscles and joint structures that could restrict hip internal rotation—primarily the psoas, short external rotators of the hip, and posterior hip capsule. As decelerators of pelvic rotation to the rear leg, the adductor longus and medial hamstrings are potential contributors to this deficit in hip internal rotation. At the ankle, a tight medial

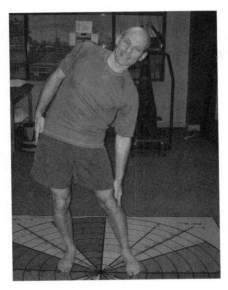

Fig. 3. Core mobility in the frontal plane.

gastrocnemius is a limiting factor in the ability to rotate the tibia externally.

(3) At the leg opposite the side of pelvic rotation, the biomechanical events of pronation occur. The relationship of the foot to the hip

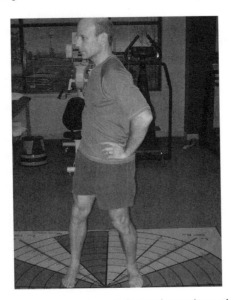

Fig. 4. Core mobility in the transverse plane. Right rotation supinates the right lower extremity and pronates the left lower extremity.

on this side is demonstrated by the ability of the subtalar joint to convert the internal rotation of the femur and tibia into calcaneal eversion [29]. Because the knee tends to flex on this side, the influence of the gastrocnemius on the subtalar joint is lessened. As a result, a restriction in calcaneal eversion and ankle dorsiflexion tends to be more articular than soft tissue related. If a lack of calcaneal eversion is seen, then manual joint techniques of the subtalar joint may be useful to improve the ability of the entire chain to absorb shock. An excessively pronated foot, where the calcaneus is everted fully to end range in weight bearing, also can be a problem.

4. Eccentric-Concentric Control of the Core (ECC): These tests look at the ability of the core muscle groups, primarily the abdominals, spinal extensors, psoas, iliacus, quadratus lumborum, latissimus dorsi, and hip girdle muscles to control the body's center of mass.

   a. Sagittal ECC (Fig. 5): This test assesses the ability of the psoas, rectus femoris, short hip adductors, and rectus abdominis to control eccentrically extension of the spine and anterior translation of the pelvis. Each side is tested. Common compensatory patterns include restricted anterior translation of the pelvis with overextension by the lumbar or thoracic spine, excessive flexion of the knee, "clawing" of the toes, or hyperactivity of the toe extensors to stabilize distally.

   b. Frontal ECC (Fig. 6): This test challenges pelvic stability in the frontal plane, which makes it an excellent test of gluteus medius function. Loss of balance or a Trendelenburg sign mark the onset of fatigue in this muscle and lateral stabilizers of the pelvis. This is a common finding, even in well-conditioned runners who train primarily in the SP, and derive minimal challenge to the FP activity of hip and thigh muscles.

   c. Transverse (Fig. 7): On the stance leg, the external abdominal oblique, contralateral internal abdominal oblique, and psoas will rotate the spine contralaterally. The gluteus maximus and deep hip rotators will rotate the pelvis contralaterally. The pelvis and spine should rotate synchronously—ipsilaterally as these muscles lengthen and contralaterally as they shorten. Motion in the spine that markedly exceeds pelvic motion in relationship to the femur of the stance leg indicates tightness in the short hip external rotators and posterior hip capsule. It also suggests an inability of the hip to load the gluteals eccentrically in the transverse plane during the propulsion stage of stance.

   d. All of these tests can be made more or less challenging to meet the functional capabilities of the runner by modifying the amount of support, speed, number of repetitions, and the range of the

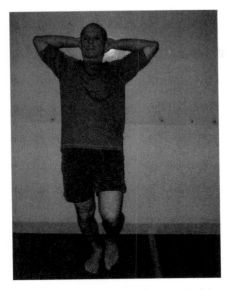

Fig. 5. Sagittal eccentric/concentric control of the core.

excursion. A successful base test requires 10 controlled repetition on each side.

5. Hip-scapula reaction (HSR): The pelvic girdle, which is connected to the scapula by the axial skeleton and associated thoracolumbar soft tissues,

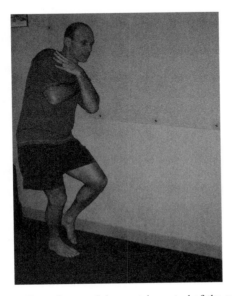

Fig. 6. Frontal eccentric/concentric control of the core.

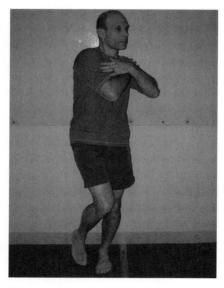

Fig. 7. Transverse eccentric/concentric control of the core.

induces a pattern of scapula motion in all three planes as a response
to its movement (Table 1). Although this "scapula reaction" is not
a mandatory movement, joint mechanics of the upper quarter are
optimized by linked movements with the trunk and pelvis. Similarly, the
mobility of the pelvis and function of the muscles of the torso and hips
are influenced by the ability of the scapula and thoracic cage to move
freely in all three planes (Figs. 8–10). In respect to running, HSR
underscores the role of the abdominals in controlling the triplanar

Table 1
Hip–shoulder relationships with hip–scapular reaction maneuvers

| Position of eccentric hip loading | Concentric hip activity | Shoulder motion | Scapula motion |
|---|---|---|---|
| I/L hip flexion | I/L hip extension | Flexion | Anterior tilt |
| C/L hip flexion | C/L hip extension | Extension | Posterior tilt |
| C/L hip internal rotation | C/L hip external rotation | External rotation | Retraction |
| I/L hip internal rotation | I/L hip external rotation | Internal rotation | Protraction |
| C/L hip adduction | C/L hip abduction | Abduction | Upward rotation |
| I/L hip adduction | I/L hip abduction | Adduction | Downward rotation |

*Abbreviations:* C/L, contralateral; I/L, ipsilateral.

movement of the spine, pelvis, and even the shoulder/arm. This controlled motion during running allows for energy-efficient movement to maintain forward momentum [30].

6. Lower extremity balance and reach: Balance and reach activities are used to accentuate the stability and mobility deficits that are noted on the squat, core, and stability tests. They also allow quantification of function by measuring the distance reached or the number of reaches that is performed in a set period of time. The direction of the reach is named by referencing the stance or balancing leg. A running-specific

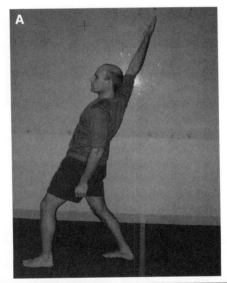

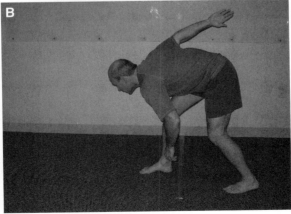

Fig. 8. Sagittal hip scapular reaction. (*A*) Shoulder flexion with ipsilateral hip extension. (*B*) Contralateral hip and shoulder extension.

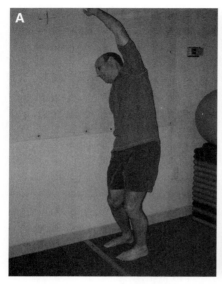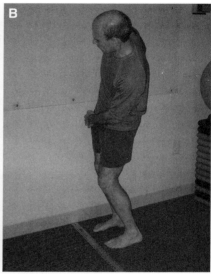

Fig. 9. Frontal hip scapular reaction. (*A*) Contralateral hip and shoulder abduction. (*B*) Shoulder adduction with ipsilateral hip abduction.

balance and reach is a bilateral upper extremity posterior overhead reach with a posterior lower limb reach. The torso should not flex to counterbalance hip extension to offset the spinal extension that is introduced by bilateral shoulder flexion (Fig. 11). This test challenges

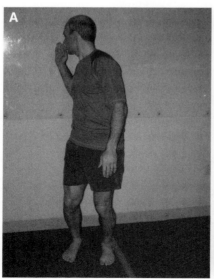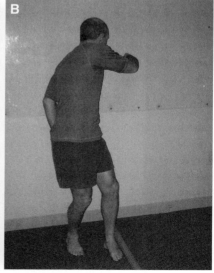

Fig. 10. Transverse hip scapular reaction. (*A*) Shoulder external rotation and ipsilateral hip internal rotation. (*B*) Shoulder internal rotation and contralateral hip internal rotation.

the runner to extend the hip without compensatory forward bending and is a functional test of the psoas' ability to lengthen eccentrically in the sagittal plane without loss of lumbar extension. This test is particularly useful when examining the runner who has hip or lumbosacral pain.

7. Open kinetic chain assessment of the foot and ankle: The examination allows assessment of the foot and ankle without the influence of soft tissues. The examiner should correlate these findings with those in the closed chain, particularly foot and ankle motion that is assessed with the single leg squat test. The following is assessed with the open kinetic chain maneuvers:

   a. Hallux dorsiflexion (first metatarsophalangeal [MTP] extension): Hallux extension of 65° to 70°, in late stance, is ideal to achieve sufficient tension in the plantar aponeurosis to lock up the foot [31] and adequate hip extension. Both are needed to perform forceful propulsion.
   b. Subtalar joint motion: With the runner seated, subtalar motion is assessed through passively inverting and everting the calcaneus. Flexion of the knee removes the influence of the gastrocnemius. An end feel assessment is made to determine if limited motion is due to a capsular/ligamentous restriction or a bony block. Because pronation is a triplanar activity of many joints and bones of the foot/ankle complex, restricted calcaneal eversion causes a cascade of

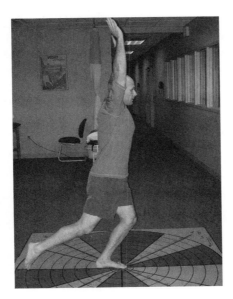

Fig. 11. Left lower extremity posterior reach with bilateral upper extremity posterior overhead reach. Movement of the limbs is referenced to the leg in stance.

events. It prevents the talus adduction and plantar flexion that is needed for loading phase after heel strike, and thus, results in a loss of dorsiflexion during midstance. A loss of ankle dorsiflexion results in restricted knee flexion and diminished sagittal plane stimulation of the quadriceps [30].

  c. Midtarsal joint motion: Midtarsal joint motion is compared in all three planes of motion with the calcaneus inverted and everted. Calcaneal eversion unlocks the midtarsal joint and makes it mobile. Conversely, calcaneal inversion restricts midtarsal motion. A midtarsal joint that does not lock with calcaneal inversion prevents shifting of body weight to the first MTP and results in an apropulsive gait or running style.

## Differential diagnosis

Overuse injuries of the hip and pelvis in runners may be classified as soft tissue injuries or as primary joint and bone pathology (Box 1). By far, in the authors' experience, soft tissue injuries are the most common in runners, particularly gluteus medius tendinopathy. Pelvis and sacroiliac joint dysfunctions are underappreciated in many clinics. In our experience, runners frequently develop superior shears, anterior innominate rotations, and sacral torsions. The diagnosis of hip labral tears, previously underappreciated in runners, is increasing in frequency as a result of better imaging with magnetic resonance arthrogram. Radicular pain in the runner also may cause hip pain. A full pattern of radiculopathy or radiculitis down the lower extremity often may not be seen. Specific evaluation techniques, such as the slump test with seated straight leg raising, is helpful in picking up radicular pain (Fig. 12). Sensitizing and relieving maneuvers with the slump test can help to differentiate hamstring tightness from adverse neurodynamic tension. Similarly, the side-lying femoral nerve stretch test uses sensitizing and relieving maneuvers and can help to differentiate quadriceps tightness from adverse neurodynamic tension in the distribution of the femoral nerve (Fig. 13).

## Treatment approaches for the runner

In the authors' experience, use of the closed kinetic chain approach is the most effective means of rehabilitating the injured runner and improving his performance because it attempts to train muscles and joints to absorb and dissipate properly the forces that are encountered in running. Closed kinetic chain exercises avoid isolating one structure in treatment; instead, this approach trains patterns of movements. In evaluation and treatment, biomechanical deficits are identified as are the planes, joints, and specific

**Box 1. Differential diagnosis of hip and pelvis overuse injuries**

*Soft tissue injuries*
  Muscle and tendon pain
    Gluteus medius tendonitis
    Hip flexor tendonitis
    Tensor fascia lata tendinitis
  Bursitis
    Trochanteric bursitis
    Ischial bursitis
  Snapping (clicking) hip
  Muscle imbalances
    Pelvic crossed syndrome
    Piriformis syndrome
  Impingement syndromes
    Anteromedial impingement
    Anterolateral impingement
    Proximal impingement
*Primary joint and bone pathology*
  Dysfunctions of the pelvis and sacroiliac joints
    Symphysis pubis
    Sacroiliac
  Joint inflammation and bony pathology
    Spondyloarthropathy, sacroiliitis, and osteitis pubis
    Stress fractures
    Avascular necrosis
    Slipped capital femoral epiphysis
    Avulsion fractures
    Coccydynia
    Osteoarthritis and hip synovitis
    Labral tears
    Tumors
*Referred pain*
  Lumbar
  Nonmusculoskeletal disorders
*Radicular pain*

activities where the runner experiences success. These activities are the basis for an initial exercise program. An understanding of the biomechanical responses that occur at each joint during pronation and supination allows the clinician to identify potential sources of injury.

Ideally, therapeutic exercise should simulate the biomechanical sequence of pronation and supination at each joint in the kinetic chain. Eccentric loading before concentric muscle contraction is a well-established approach

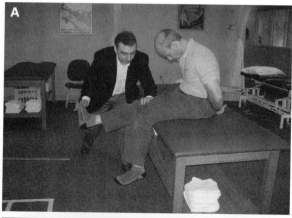

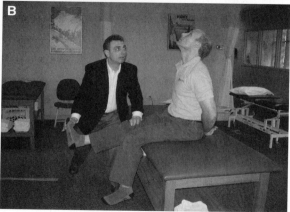

Fig. 12. Slump test. (*A*) Sensitizing maneuvers: introduction of knee extension and neck flexion. (*B*) Relieving maneuvers: introduction of head and neck extension.

for facilitating weak and inhibited muscles [32], such as with plyometrics. During the acute phase, therapeutic closed kinetic chain positions provide ways to train muscles to decelerate forces within functional ranges of motion, without causing further overload. Controlled eccentric lengthening also plays a role in treating tight muscles. Isolated stretching of tight muscles can be minimized if they are trained to lengthen eccentrically during functional activity.

The authors have found that a closed kinetic chain approach, which is based on the following principles, to be useful for safe and early mobilization:

The symptomatic and overloaded structure should not be the initial site of treatment. Faulty biomechanics elsewhere in the kinetic chain can be addressed first.

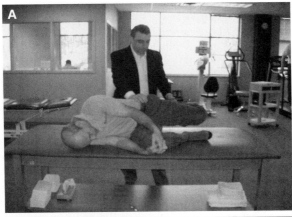

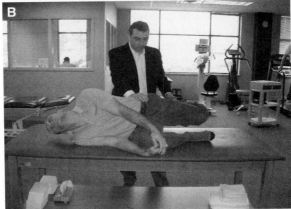

Fig. 13. Femoral nerve tension test. (*A*) Sensitizing maneuvers: introduction of knee flexion and neck flexion. (*B*) Relieving maneuver: introduction of head and neck extension.

All muscles have three planes of action. Motion that is not tolerated in one plane may be tolerated in the other two without threat of tissue overload.

All muscles are potential synergists to each other. Improving the ability of the gastroc-soleus to lengthen eccentrically with the subtalar joint inverted, as occurs at the end of stance phase, improves the ability to extend the hip. This eccentrically loads the psoas muscle to prepare it for concentric contraction in swing phase.

Closed kinetic chain activities often are tolerated better than open kinetic chain activities. Joint compression forces are reduced with closed chain proprioceptive neuromuscular facilitation exercises because it stimulates cocontraction of the muscles around the joint and make it more stable [32].

*Common conditions and treatment approaches*

*Sacroiliac and innominate dysfunction*

It is beyond the scope of this article to describe the diagnostic criteria and treatment of the 14 mechanical dysfunctions of the pelvis that were described by Greenman [33]. These respond well to muscle energy technique or high velocity low amplitude thrust. Exercise that reinforces the manual correction is necessary to prevent dependence on passive manipulative treatment. Lambert [34] developed a simplified classification of pelvic and sacral instability that is based on innominate and sacroiliac function in gait or running. The innominates demonstrate instability anteriorly or superiorly, but not posteriorly because the pelvis in gait does not rotate posteriorly beyond neutral in the sagittal plane. The sacrum flexes and rotates to the opposite side relative to the anterior leg and extends and rotates to the same side relative to the posterior leg. An exercise to mobilize the sacrum and pelvis relies on a stride position and diagonal patterns of the upper extremities (Fig. 14). Many of the same principles that are discussed below regarding treatment of causative biomechanical problems of the soft tissues of the pelvis are applicable to treatment of recurrent sacroiliac and innominate dysfunction.

*Capsular and joint dysfunction of the hip*

Restriction of hip motion that is noted on the core mobility examination can be confirmed, if necessary, with a joint play examination of the hip. A hard restricted capsular end feel is an indication for mobilization. The portions of the hip capsule that are tight can be mobilized manually using joint play techniques [33] or in functional positions that allow the additional mobilizing force of the patient's body weight and direction of movement. The pattern of correction can be carried over into a functional exercise (Fig. 15). The treatment of muscle imbalance that is associated with hip joint dysfunction is described below.

*Overload of soft tissues*

The runner who presents with hip tendonitis or strain usually has a history of a change in running surface or intensity, most often an increase in mileage. The primary disrupting force is repetitive tensile forces that result in microtrauma.

Initial management of muscle strains and tendonitis consists of ice, compression, and decreased weight bearing. Relative rest is a key concept to follow to avoid needless immobilization. Pain-free motion is allowed in planes that are not disruptive to the injury and at joints that are biomechanically linked to the affected area. Initially, eccentric loading is avoided. It is introduced gradually, as tissue repair proceeds, to minimize the chance of tissue disruption. In the latter stages of rehabilitation, rapidly applied eccentric loads are used to develop tensile strength at the

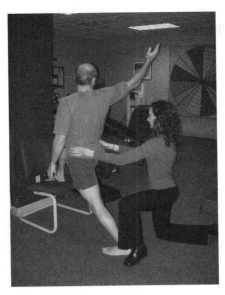

Fig. 14. Self-mobilization of the right sacral base restricted in extension and right rotation.

musculotendinous junction and at osseotendinous insertions to train the muscle to decelerate loads [35].

A closed kinetic chain paradigm of rehabilitation is presented below for the hamstrings. The basic premise of this approach, establishing and

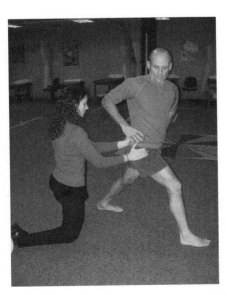

Fig. 15. Functional mobilization of the right posterior hip capsule in a stride position.

treating causative biomechanical sources of dysfunction, are applicable to soft tissue injury elsewhere in the pelvis.

The hamstrings are subjected to high tensile load given their extensive eccentric role in running. During initial swing, the knee and hip are flexing which requires simultaneous eccentric and concentric activity of the hamstrings. During the last portion of swing, the hamstrings continue to play a dual role—controlling knee extension while extending the hip. The hamstrings work synergistically with the gluteals to stabilize, decelerate, and propel the hip in running [36]. During the propulsion phase, the medial hamstrings assist in decelerating hip external rotation. This maintains the gluteus maximus at an ideal length to act as an accelerator, along with the hamstrings, of the femur in the sagittal plane. The hamstrings, along with the rectus abdominis, also are decelerators of pelvic anterior tilt throughout stance. Given these functional relationships, it is conceivable that hamstring strain or rupture has its source in the inhibition and weakness of its closest synergists, the gluteals and abdominals [37].

It is the authors' opinion that function of the foot and ankle and scapulothoracic region has a direct bearing on muscle facilitation and inhibition of the trunk and hip. These relationships were described in the section on functional evaluation. Thus, the first step in treating muscle imbalance of the hip, regardless of the affected tissue, is to correct the biomechanical deficits of the foot and ankle that are the source of altered gait mechanics. As well, improving the mobility of the scapula and thoracic spine facilitates eccentric stimulation of the abdominals and enhances their role as pelvic stabilizers.

Hamstring retraining following the initial phase of repair starts with identifying pain-free planes of motion. Often, the hamstring can be loaded in the TP or FP using an approach that combines reaches of the upper extremity with pelvic translation. Ultimately, the hamstring must be able to handle high tensile loads, primarily in the SP, for a successful return to running [38].

Regardless of the soft tissue or joint that is injured, a milestone in the rehabilitation of the runner is the ability to control higher eccentric loads in asymptomatic planes. Closed kinetic chain loading of a muscle can be increased by using steps of different heights, displacing the body's center of mass, or adding external weight. The ability to control body weight for 10 repetitions graduates the runner to a more challenging exercise in the same plane and allow for the introduction of activities with lighter loads in previously symptomatic planes of motion. The optimal exercise cadence of eccentric to concentric muscle contraction for strengthening is 3:1 (6-second eccentric to 2-second concentric) at the maximum weight that can be controlled for 10 repetitions [39]. Once strength in a specific plane is no longer an issue, rehabilitation can focus on power training at functional speeds with a lighter load. The goal is to be able to perform strength and power exercises in all three planes of motion asymptomatically or with minimal symptoms at higher loads. At this point, rehabilitation of the runner begins to transition into performance training.

*Returning to running and performance training for running*

A graded program of walking and running is instrumental for correcting specific biomechanical problems and meeting the runner's psychologic need to return to his sport quickly. Running is an SP-dominant activity, but relies on muscles to provide triplanar stability and mobility at the pelvis with each stride. Use of walking and running stride patterns that incorporate TP and FP motion of the arms and trunk; frequent changes in the direction of progression; or changing the base of support are useful for training hip girdle muscles that primarily function in planes other than the SP. As a tool in rehabilitation, walking or running other than "straight ahead" may be tolerated better than conventional walking or "slow jogging." This approach can be used with cross-training to help maintain the runner's cardiovascular fitness. The runner should be encouraged to continue this form of walking and running as a warm-up and cool-down, and, whenever possible in a training run, to include these patterns of motion to keep muscles and joints active in multiple planes of motion.

Returning to running after a hip or pelvic injury requires an incremental increase in mileage and speed. A protocol by James [40] for returning to running following injury is based on missed running time. Injuries that result in at least 4 weeks of missed training require approximately 9 weeks of a combined walking and running program before the runner can return to previous training levels. A "walk to run program" [41] proposes a regimen that incorporates walking and running over a 12-week period with an increasing proportion of running relative to walking each successive week. Speed and mileage progression should be based on the runner's symptoms. Loss of bone density is a concern following a prolonged layoff from running. Therefore, an incremental progression in intensity and mileage is required to prevent stress fracture. Ideally, rehabilitation of the runner should incorporate exercises that stimulate an increase in bone density. A simple regimen of heel drops, performed at a frequency of 50 repetitions per day, increased hip and spine bone density by 3% to 4% [42].

There is no shortage of training myths and unsound training practices in running. A common misconception is that running is sufficient to increase leg strength. Hennessy and Watson [43] found that endurance training that consisted of moderate running 4 days a week for 30 minutes to 60 minutes did not improve leg strength as measured by squat testing. In the same study, a group of athletes that used strength training improved their leg strength and speed and also maintained their endurance. The need to include strength training in the athlete's training regimen after injury should be appreciated in light of the observations of Nadler et al [44] that kinetic chain functional deficits persist long after recovery from an injury.

The role of stretching for improving performance and avoiding injury is overestimated. A recent review of the literature by Thacker et al [16] found no evidence in the randomized controlled trials that stretching alone prevents injury. The investigators recommended a comprehensive program of warm-up, including stretching and conditioning exercises. Tolerance of a rapidly applied eccentric load, which can result in strain, may be the key point for preventing muscle injury. The relationship of muscle injury and muscle flexibility may be more a function of the length at which the muscle develops peak torque, rather than its ability to elongate passively [45]. It is in this respect that eccentric overloading in training plays an important role in preventing soft tissue injury at the hip. Askling et al [46] found that in male elite soccer players, eccentric training of the hamstrings that was performed once or twice per week for 10 weeks resulted in significantly less hamstring strains and increased speed and strength when compared with a matched group that did not receive this training. Appendix A describes a functional progression for injury prevention and performance enhancement that emphasizes the eccentric role of muscle activity in running.

In summary, resistance training can be used to improve running performance. This type of program can be tailored to meet the entire spectrum of performance goals from power training for sprinters to endurance training for marathoners. The common denominator from the early stage of rehabilitation to performance training is the use of a triplanar closed kinetic chain approach. The authors have found this to be the best way to prepare the hip and the entire kinetic chain for the specific demands of running.

**Summary**

The runner is especially at risk for development of injury to the hip and pelvis secondary to chronic repetitive microtrauma. The key to treatment is establishing complete and accurate diagnosis, and, in particular, identifying the functional biomechanical deficits in the kinetic chain that contribute to this repetitive microtrauma.

A long-term successful outcome and prevention of reinjury are more likely if the focus of rehabilitation is on the restoration of the functional kinetic chain, rather than on a specific injured tissue. For example, the typical treatment of "iliotibial band syndrome" is a stretching protocol that frequently is unsuccessful in the long-term improvement of symptoms. A functional biomechanical approach might identify that the injured runner has lack of calcaneal eversion and a structurally rigid supinated foot. These functional biomechanical deficits would lead to inadequate internal rotation of the tibia and femur and result in inhibition or decreased recruitment of the gluteal muscles, in particular the gluteus medius. Restoring pronation throughout the lower extremity would require joint play techniques or functional joint mobilizations for the foot and ankle. In addition, a running shoe with a cushioned heel may be necessary to promote pronation and to attenuate shock. Exercises that integrate foot and hip function, including balance reaches, lunges and step-downs, are prescribed to stimulate the gluteus medius and other gluteals in positions that simulate running. Activities that are done in this manner activate the entire functional kinetic chain of muscles and joints.

The nonoperative sports medicine specialist, in particular the physiatrist and physical therapist, are in an excellent position to integrate treatment of the entire functional kinetic chain through a thorough biomechanical evaluation and comprehensive rehabilitation of the injured runner. Additional training in the areas of biomechanical evaluation and functional biomechanical deficits should be sought, because residency and even many fellowship-trained programs often overlook these important areas.

Finally, the injured runner is best taken care of in a setting in which different sports medicine specialists are available and work well as a team. No one sports medicine specialist can provide all of the needs to the injured runner.

## Appendix A

Functional Progression for Performance Enhancement and Injury Prevention
I. Combined Stretching and Strengthening
A. Squat Progression–Technique is head and chest up, neutral or extended spine, and hips translated posteriorly.
1. Two-legged on stable surface–20 reps (Figure 16)
2. Two-legged on unstable (wobble board or disco-sits) surface–10 reps (Figure 17)
3. One-legged on stable surface–10 reps (Figure 18)
4. One-legged on unstable surface–5 reps (Figure 19)
All above squats are done with good technique, to fatigue, working up to specified repetitions.
B. Balance/reach with progression to step-downs.
1. May be done in one of three planes at 6 second eccentric/2 second concentric phases to build strength the fastest [39].
a. Anterior (Figure 20)
b. Medial (Figure 21)
c. Posteromedial rotational (Figure 22)
Works whole lower extremity by 3D stretching and strengthening.
C. Balance/reach in step-downs with bilateral upper extremity (UE) 3-D reaches for integrated core, scapulo-thoracic, and lower extremities (LE).

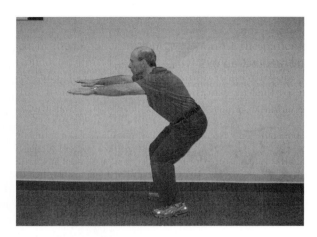

Fig. 16. Bilateral squat—stable surface.

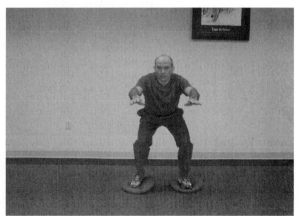

Fig. 17. Bilateral squat—unstable surface.

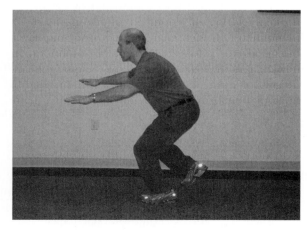

Fig. 18. Unilateral squat—stable surface.

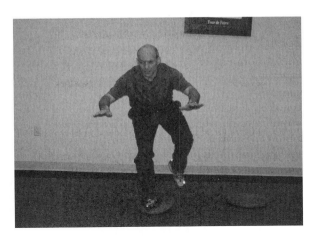

Fig. 19. Unilateral squat—unstable surface.

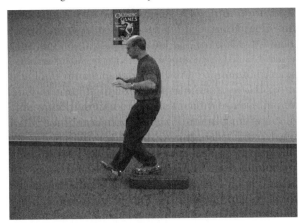

Fig. 20. Anterior step-down.

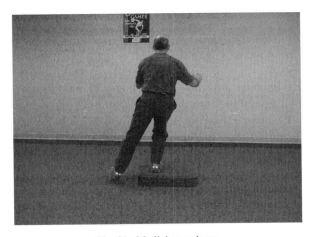

Fig. 21. Medial step-down.

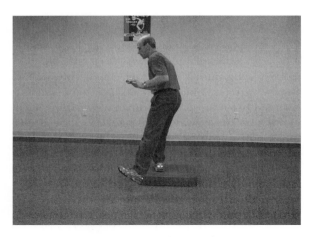

Fig. 22. Posteromedial step-down.

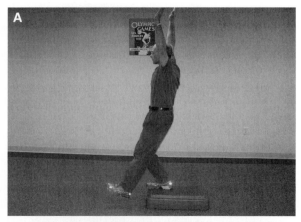

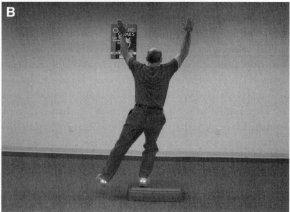

Fig. 23. (*A*) Anterior step-down with bilateral upper limb overhead reach. (*B*) Medial step-down with bilateral upper limb overhead reach. (*C*) Posteromedial step-down with bilateral upper limb overhead reach.

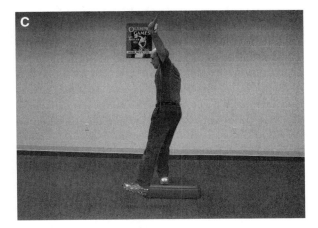

Fig. 23 (*continued*)

1. Above three balance and reach and/or step-downs maneuvers combined with:
a. Bilateral overhead UE reaches (Figures 23 a–c)
b. Bilateral overhead/sidebending UE reaches (Figures 24 a–c)
c. Bilateral rotational UE reaches at hip height (Figures 25 a–c)
d. 3-D lunges with UE 3D stretches (Figures 26–29 a–c)
1) Dynamically stretches and strengthens LE and core musculature.
D. Landing drills for eccentric control of initial landing phase of running (from 2"-8"). All done with slow eccentric (6 second phase)
1. Bilateral jump-downs
2. Unilateral hop-downs
Above two exercises with combined 3-D UE reaches at hip, shoulder, and overhead heights at this frequency and intensity of the 3-D functional exercises:
a. Frequency
1) Injury Recovery Phase:
(a) Runner is walking, but not running yet.
(b) Minimum 2 and maximum 3 times a week.
2) Walk/Run Phase:
(a) 2 times per week.
3) Peak Running Performance Phase
(a) 1 time per week.
(b) 4–5 days per week of running.
(c) 1–2 days per week of rest, depending on age and responses to this training program.
b. Intensity
1) Intrinsic Weight:
(a) Body weight and gravity.

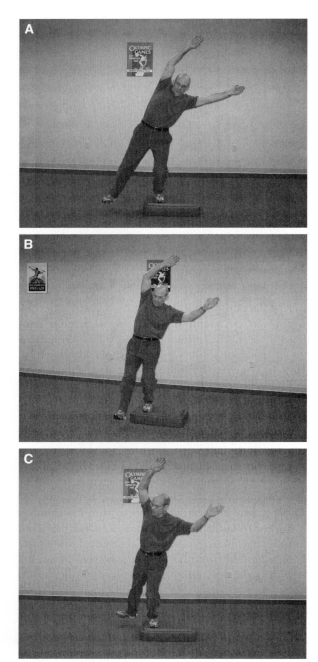

Fig. 24. (*A*) Anterior step-down with bilateral upper limb side-bending reach. (*B*) Medial step-down with bilateral upper limb side-bending reach. (*C*) Posteromedial step-down with bilateral upper limb side-bending reach.

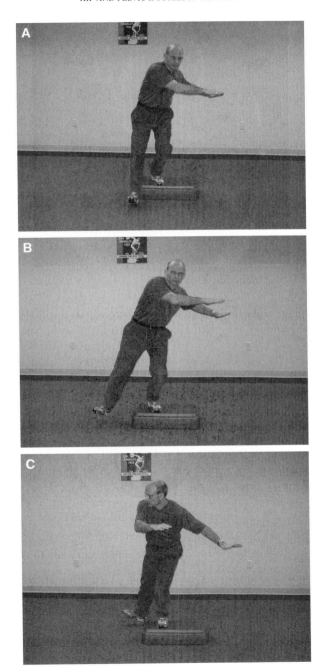

Fig. 25. (*A*) Anterior step-down with bilateral upper limb rotational reach. (*B*) Medial step-down with bilateral upper limb rotational reach. (*C*) Posteromedial step-down with bilateral upper limb rotational reach.

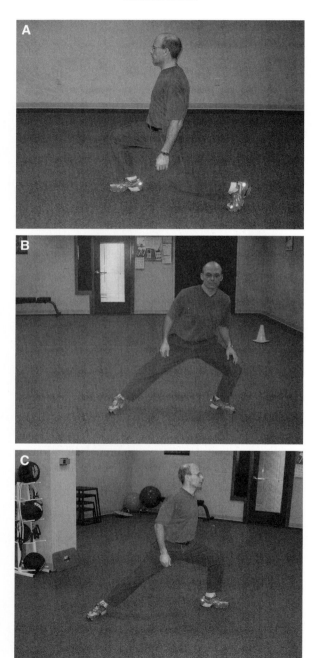

Fig. 26. (*A*) Anterior lunge. (*B*) Lateral lunge. (*C*) Posterolateral rotational lunge.

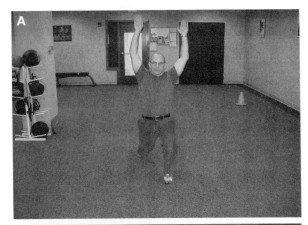

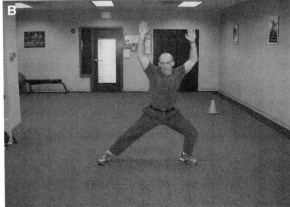

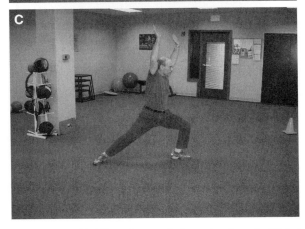

Fig. 27. (*A*) Anterior lunge with bilateral upper limb overhead reach. (*B*) Lateral lunge with bilateral upper limb overhead reach. (*C*) Posterolateral rotation lunge with bilateral upper limb overhead reach.

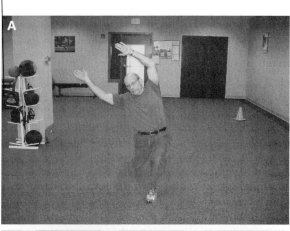

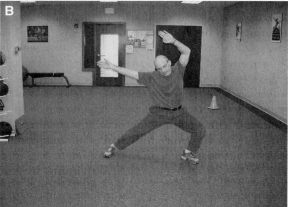

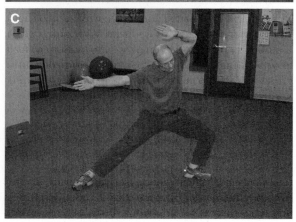

Fig. 28. (*A*) Anterior lunge with bilateral upper limb side-bending reach. (*B*) Lateral lunge with bilateral upper limb side-bending reach. (*C*) Posterolateral rotational lunge with bilateral upper limb side-bending reach.

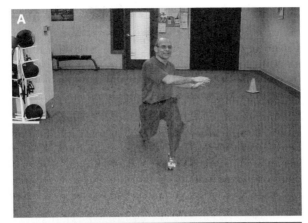

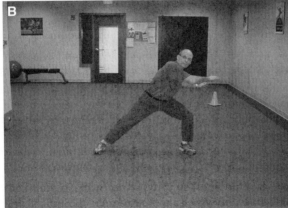

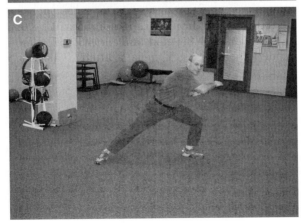

Fig. 29. (*A*) Anterior lunge with bilateral upper limb rotational reach. (*B*) Lateral lunge with bilateral upper limb rotational reach. (*C*) Posterolateral lunge with bilateral upper limb rotational reach.

(b) Extrinsic weight: barbells, dumbbells, medicine and kettle balls, weighted vest, etc.

(c) Strength progression guidelines:
    –8–10 reps
    –Increased weight when good control and technique can be performed
    –Start with 60–80% of 1 $rep_{max}$

(d) Endurance progression: 20–25 reps with increasing speed at 10–15% of 1 $rep_{max}$.

## References

[1] Lloyd-Smith R, Clement DB, McKenzie DC, et al. A survey of overuse and traumatic hip and pelvis injuries in athletes. Phys Sportsmed 1995;13:131–41.

[2] Geraci MC. Rehabilitation of pelvis, hip and thigh injures in sports. Phys Med Rehabil Clin N Am 1994;5:157–73.

[3] Hreljac A. Evaluation of lower extremity overuse injury potential in runners. Med Sci Sports Exerc 1999;32:1635–41.

[4] Marti B, Vader JP, Minder CE, et al. On the epidemiology of running injuries: the 1984 Bern Grand-Prix study. Am J Sports Med 1988;16:285–93.

[5] Rolf C. Overuse injuries of the lower extremity in runners. Scand J Med Sci Sports 1995; 5:181–90.

[6] Van Mechelen W. Can running injuries be effectively prevented? Sports Med 1995;19:161–5.

[7] Beckman SM, Buchanan TS. Ankle inversion injury and hypermobility: effect of hip and ankle muscle electromyography onset latency. Arch Phys Med Rehabil 1995;76(12): 1138–43.

[8] Vleeming A, Stoekart R, Volkers ACW, et al. Relationships between form and function in the sacroiliac joint. Part II: biomechanical aspects. Spine 1990;15:133–5.

[9] Bowen V, Cassidy JD. Macroscopic and microscopic anatomy of the sacroiliac joint from embryonic life until the eight decade. Spine 1981;6:620–8.

[10] Jull GA, Janda V. Muscles and motor control in low back pain: assessment and management. In: Twomey LT, Taylor JR, editors. Physical therapy of the low back. Clinics in physical therapy. New York: Churchill Livingstone; 1987. p. 253–78.

[11] Vleeming A, Stoeckart R, Volkers ACW, et al. Relationship between form and function in the sacroiliac joint. Part I: clinical anatomical aspects. Spine 1990;15:130–2.

[12] Vleeming A, Stoeckart R, Volkers ACW, et al. Relationship between form and function in the sacroiliac joint. Part II: biomechanical aspects. Spine 1990;15:133–5.

[13] Vleeming A, Stoeckart R, Snijders CJ. The sacrotuberous ligament: a conceptual approach to its dynamic role in stabilizing the sacroiliac joint. Clin Biomech (Bristol, Avon) 1989;4: 201–3.

[14] Colachis SC, Worden RE, Bechtol CO, Strohm BR. Movements of the sacroiliac joint in the adult male. Arch Phys Med Rehabil 1963;44:490–8.

[15] Egund N, Olsson TH, Schmid H, et al. Movements in the sacroiliac joints demonstrated with roentgen stereophotogrammetry. Acta Radiol 1978;19:833–46.

[16] Thacker SB, Gilchrist J, Stroup DF, et al. The impact of stretching on sports injury risk: a systematic review of the literature. MSSE 2003;36:371–8.

[17] McGill S. Ultimate back fitness and performance. Waterloo, Canada: Wabuno Publishers; 2004.

[18] Gray GW. Pronation and supination. Available at: http://www.functionaldesign.com/ wynn_marketing/newsarticles. Accessed September 29, 2004.

[19] Pearson KG. Generating the walking gait: role of sensory feedback. Prog Brain Res 2004; 143:123–9.

[20] Van Den Bogert A, Read L, Nigg B. An analysis of hip joint loading during walking, running and skiing. Med Sci Sports Exerc 1999;31(1):131–42.

[21] Anderson K, Strickland SM, Warren R. Hip and groin injuries in athletes. Am J Sports Med 2001;29:521–33.

[22] Hreljac A, Marshall RN, Hume PA. Evaluation of lower extremity overuse injury potential in runners. Med Sci Sports Exerc 2003;32(9):1635–41.

[23] Hreljac A. Impact and overuse injuries in runners. Med Sci Sports Exerc 2004;36(5):845–9.

[24] Lun V, Meeuwisse WH, Stergiou P, Stefanyshyn D. Relation between running injury and static lower limb alignment in recreational runners. Br J Sports Med 2004;38(5):576–80.

[25] Williams DS III, Davis IM, Scholz JP, et al. High-arched runners exhibit increased leg stiffness compared to low-arched runners. Gait Posture 2004;19(3):263–9.

[26] Furman University. Biomechanics of running and body composition. Available at: http://alpha.furman.edu/academics/dept/hes/FIRST_BIOMECHANICAL_RUNNING.pdf. Accessed September 29, 2004.

[27] Ferber R, Davis IM, Williams DS III. Gender differences in lower extremity mechanics during running. Clin Biomech (Bristol, Avon) 2003;18(4):350–7.

[28] Tiberio D, Gray GW. Kinematics and kinetics during gait. In: Donatelli R, Wooden MJ, editors. Orthopaedic physical therapy. New York: Churchill Livingstone; 1989. p. 305–20.

[29] Inman VT. The joints of the ankle. Baltimore (MD): Williams and Wilkins; 1976.

[30] Gray GW. Running-more than just fast walking. Adrian (MI): Functional Design Systems. Functional Video Digest 2003;2(7).

[31] Donatelli R. Normal anatomy and biomechanics. In: Donatelli R, Wolf S, editors. The biomechanics of the foot and ankle. Philadelphia: F.A. Davis Company; 1990. p. 3–31.

[32] Sullivan P, Markos P, Minor MD. An integrated approach to therapeutic exercise: theory & clinical application. Reston (VA): Reston Publishing Company; 1982.

[33] Greenman P. Principles of manual medicine. 2nd edition. Baltimore (MD): Williams and Wilkins; 1996.

[34] Lambert M. Functional mobilization of the sacrum, innominates, spine and ribs. Course syllabus June 2002.

[35] Humble RN, Nugent IL. Achilles tendonitis. An overview and reconditioning model. Clin Podiatr Med Surg 2001;18(2):233–54.

[36] Norkin CC, Levangie PK. Joint structure and function: a comprehensive analysis. 2nd edition. Philadelphia: F.A. Davis Company; 1992.

[37] Geraci MC Jr. Overuse injuries of the hip and pelvis. J Back Musculoskeletal Rehabil 1996; 6:5–19.

[38] Gray GW, Tiberio D. Chain reaction explosion. Precourse video. Available at: http://www.functionaldesign.com. Accessed March 23, 2005.

[39] Evans WJ, Couzens GC. Astrofit: the astronaut program for anti-aging. New York: Simon and Schuster; 2002.

[40] James SL. Running injuries of the knee. Instr Course Lect 1998;47:407–17.

[41] Hamilton J. Walk to run. Available at: http://www.runningstrong.com. Accessed August 1, 2004.

[42] Bassey EJ. Exercise for the prevention of osteoporotic fracture. Age Aging 2001;4:29–31.

[43] Hennessy LC, Watson AWS. The interference effects of training for strength and endurance simultaneously. J Strength Cond Res 1994;8(1):12–9.

[44] Nadler SF, Malanga GA, Feinberg JM, Rubanni M, Moley P, Foye P. Functional performance deficits in athletes with previous lower extremity injury. Clin J Sport Med 2002; 12(2):73–8.

[45] Brockett C, Morgan D, Proske U. Predicting hamstring strain in elite athletes. Med Sci Sports Exerc 2004;36(3):379–87.

[46] Askling C, Karlsson J, Thorstensson A. Hamstring injury occurrence in elite soccer players after preseason strength training with eccentric overload. Scand J Med Sci Sports 2003;13(4): 244–50.

ELSEVIER
SAUNDERS

Phys Med Rehabil Clin N Am
16 (2005) 749–777

PHYSICAL MEDICINE
AND REHABILITATION
CLINICS OF
NORTH AMERICA

# Stress Fractures and Knee Injuries
# in Runners

Anne Z. Hoch, DO, PT[a],*, Michelle Pepper, MD[b],
Venu Akuthota, MD[c]

[a]Department of Orthopaedic Surgery, Medical College of Wisconsin, Froedtert East Clinics,
Fifth Floor, 9200 West Wisconsin Avenue, Milwaukee, WI 53226, USA
[b]Medical College of Wisconsin, 9200 West Wisconsin Avenue, Milwaukee, WI 53226, USA
[c]Department of Physical Medicine and Rehabilitation University of Colorado School of
Medicine, P.O. Box 6510, Mail Stop F721, Aurora, CO 80045, USA

The increase of athletics in the lives of women has been muted by their rate of lower limb musculoskeletal injury. Stress fractures and knee overuse injuries, in particular, have become epidemic in female running athletes. The putative "female athlete triad" and subsequent bone demineralization has led to higher rates of stress fractures among women. Knee injuries, including patellofemoral pain and iliotibial band syndrome, are extremely common in sports medicine and occur with a much higher incidence in female runners. These entities are discussed in detail in this following article.

## Stress fractures

### Bone basic science

Injury to bone encompasses an array of defects of bone architecture from bone strain to stress reaction to nondisplaced stress fracture to displaced fracture. Essentially, these injuries occur when bone fails to remodel adequately with the application of repetitive subthreshold stress. Because running and jogging involve ground reaction forces that are three to eight times greater than walking, distance runners and track athletes are particularly prone to developing stress fractures.

An understanding of bone basic science is needed to illuminate the etiologies and treatment principles for stress fractures. Bone is a highly organized and dynamic living tissue with metabolic and structural

* Corresponding author.
E-mail address: azeni@mcw.edu (A.Z. Hoch).

1047-9651/05/$ - see front matter © 2005 Elsevier Inc. All rights reserved.
doi:10.1016/j.pmr.2005.02.008                                        pmr.theclinics.com

components. These components are interdependent and responsive to each other. The metabolic component involves mineral homeostasis and bone remodeling, whereas the structural component involves maintaining skeletal integrity and bone remodeling.

At the microscopic level, bone has two forms, woven and lamellar. Woven bone is an immature type that is found in the embryo and newborn; lamellar bone is more mature bone and, through remodeling, replaces woven bone by 4 years of age [1]. It is more highly organized, with stress-oriented collagen that makes it anisotropic (mechanical properties differ depending on the direction of applied force) [2].

Normal lamellar bone is organized structurally into cortical (compact) bone or cancellous (trabecular) bone. Cortical bone makes up 80% of the skeleton and is composed of tightly packed osteons or haversian system. Osteons usually are oriented in the long axis of the bone and are connected by haversian canals [3]. Cortical bone is found principally at the diaphysis of long bones and the shell of cuboidlike bones, such as vertebral bodies or tarsal and carpal bones. Cortical bone is characterized by eight times slower metabolic turnover compared with cancellous bone and four times greater mass. Most stress fractures in runners occur in cortical bone (Box 1).

Cancellous (trabecular) bone is found principally at the metaphysis and epiphysis of long bones and in cuboidlike bones. It is less dense and undergoes more stress remodeling. Clinically, bone mineral density (BMD) studies measure areas that contain mostly cancellous bone (vertebral bodies, femoral trochanter, and sacrum) because of its earlier/greater rate of bone turnover and its greater likelihood of demonstrating a change in BMD.

There are three major types of bone cells: osteoblasts, osteocytes, and osteoclasts. Osteoblasts are derived from undifferentiated mesenchymal cells. They line the surface of bones and function primarily to produce bone matrix (type I collagen and osteocalcin). Osteoblasts have receptors for parathyroid hormone (PTH) and 1,25-dihydroxyvitamin D [1,4]. In general, these hormones function systemically by way of an osteoblastic mediator. PTH directly inhibits osteoblastic formation of osteocalcin, whereas 1,25-dihydroxyvitamin D stimulates osteocalcin formation. Locally, an osteoblast is stimulated by several growth factors, including transforming growth factor–β-1, -2, and -3; bone morphogenic proteins 1–7; insulin-like growth factors I and II; and acidic and basic fibroblast growth factor [1,4].

---

**Box 1. Frequent sites of stress fractures in runners (by order of incidence)**

Tibia
Metatarsal
Fibula
Navicular

Osteocytes are former osteoblasts that have become surrounded with bone mineral matrix (calcified bone). Osteocytes function to maintain bone and control extracellular concentrations of calcium and phosphorus. The final cell type, osteoclasts, is derived from hematopoietic precursors and function to resorb bone. They bind to the bone surface and resorb an isolated area of bone by dissolving the hydroxyapatite crystals and digesting the collagen. Osteoclasts have specific receptors for calcitonin and, when bound, calcitonin directly inhibits bone resorption. Osteoclasts do not have receptors for PTH or 1,25-dihydroxyvitamin D, and therefore, are stimulated indirectly by these hormones through an osteoblast-mediated mechanism to increase bone resorption [1].

The macroscopic composition of bone differs depending on site, age, diet, and disease. In general, the mineral or inorganic phase accounts for 60% of the tissue, the organic phase accounts for 35%, and water accounts for the remaining 5%. The mineral or inorganic phase consists of crystalline calcium hydroxyapatite $(Ca_{10}(PO_4)_6(OH)_2)$. It is responsible for the compressive strength of bone. The organic phase consists of 90% type I collagen and is responsible for the tensile strength of bone. The remainder of the organic phase consists of proteoglycans, matrix proteins, growth factors, and cytokines.

In general, the expected age of peak bone mass accrual is between 25 and 30 years [4]. After this age, men and women gradually lose bone mass. Girls seem to acquire most of their bone mass at an earlier age than boys (age 11–14 years compared with 13–17 years) [4,5]. Women who are postmenopausal or hypoestrogenic for other reasons have accelerated bone loss that is due to increased bone resorption compared with formation. Therefore, female athletes who are hypoestrogenic during adolescence can accrue a lower peak bone mass, which might be an irreversible problem after a certain age [4,6,7]. Using bone turnover markers, it was observed that amenorrheic runners have a reduced bone turnover, especially in bone formation, compared with eumenorrheic runners. This is believed to be linked to the various endocrine abnormalities (including hypoestrogenemia), low body mass index, and low energy intake relative to expenditure [8]. Recent studies suggest that the altered energy balance ultimately may cause this imbalance in bone homeostasis. Chronic undernutrition and acute dietary energy restriction are accompanied by reduced bone formation. The latter also has been associated with depressed levels of insulin-like growth factor 1, a hormone that was shown to stimulate the production of type I collagen [9–11]. Uncoupling of bone formation and resorption can be seen with restricted energy availability as little as 126 kJ/kg of lean body mass/d [12].

*Bone remodeling*

According to Wolff's Law, bone has a cellular and molecular remodeling response to applied mechanical stress. The bony adaptation is a function of the number of loading cycles, cycle frequency, amount of strain, strain rate, and strain duration per cycle [13]. Cortical and cancellous bone remodel continuously by osteoclastic and osteoblastic activity. This remodeling occurs throughout life and is affected by multiple factors, including metabolic state, nutritional status, menstrual patterns, age, sex, level of fitness, and ethnicity. Bone also responds to piezoelectric changes. Tensile forces create electropositivity, and thereby, stimulate osteoclastic activity [13]. Compressive forces create electronegativity, and thereby, stimulate osteoblastic activity. Most cortical stresses in nature are tension. Torsion or twisting provides tension circumferentially, whereas bending produces tension on the convex side and compression on the concave side. Tension forces were shown to result in microfracture and debonding at cement lines [14].

Clinically, this concept becomes important in the treatment of femoral neck stress fractures. Compression-side injuries (on the medial inferior cortex of the femoral neck) heal much better than traction-side stress injuries (on the lateral superior cortex of the femoral neck). Because of their robust ability to heal, nondisplaced compression-type stress fractures typically are treated with nonweight bearing until the patient becomes pain-free, which may take several days to weeks. Tension-type femoral neck stress fractures may fail to heal adequately with serious sequela, such as avascular necrosis, malunion or nonunion, or varus deformity. Thus, tension- side fractures often require internal fixation.

*Stress injury*

Stress injury occurs on a continuum from normal bone remodeling and repair to frank cortical fracture. Overall bone health depends on mechanical, hormonal, nutritional, and genetic factors. The susceptibility of bone to fracture under fluctuating stresses is related to the crystal structure and collagen orientation of the osteon. Fatigue load under certain strain rates can cause progressive accumulation of microdamage [15]. When such a process is prolonged, bone eventually may fail through crack propagation. Bone simultaneously repairs these cracks by new bone formation at their tips, and thereby, decreases the chance for propagation.

Stress injury of bone is the result of excessive bone strain with accumulation of microdamage and inability to keep up with appropriate skeletal repair (fatigue reaction/fracture), or depressed bony remodeling in response to normal strain (insufficiency reaction/fracture). The former situation most likely occurs in athletes and military recruits. The latter most likely occurs with the female athlete triad, metabolic bone disease, and osteoporosis. Sacral insufficiency stress fractures have been found to occur in female runners and often mimic the presentation of sacroiliitis. There also may be a component of reperfusion injury following prolonged strenuous exercise that results in bone tissue ischemia. This may help to explain how some stress fractures occur in cortical bone areas of lower strain and when intracortical osteopenia precedes evidence of microscopic cracks [16].

An additional consideration in the athletic population is training regimens and stress injury. Muscles exert a protective effect on cortical bone by acting as the major shock absorber. With muscle contraction, cortical bone surface bending strains are reduced [17,18]. In most weight-bearing bones it is believed that with muscle fatigue, the shock-absorbing effect is lessened and more force is transmitted directly to bone which increases the likelihood of microdamage accumulation. In nonweight-bearing and some weight-bearing bones, repetitive contraction of the muscle at its insertion may generate enough force to cause stress-induced injury [19].

## Etiology of stress fractures

Numerous factors contribute to the risk of stress fractures in runners, particularly female athletes; however, many of these proposed etiologies remain unproven. Much of the research that investigates stress fracture risks has been done in male subjects and military recruits; therefore, findings may not necessarily be generalized to female athletic populations. Furthermore, many risk factors for stress fractures are interrelated and methodologically are difficult to analyze independently.

The etiology of stress fractures is multifactorial; individual athletes vary in their susceptibility to stress injury. Risk factors (Box 2) are divided into extrinsic (characteristics of the environment in which the athlete trains or competes) and intrinsic (characteristics of the athlete herself) types.

### Extrinsic risk factors

*Training regimen.* High training volume is a major risk factor in stress fracture development. Multiple studies in runners demonstrated that higher weekly running mileage correlates with increased incidence of stress fractures [20] and overall running injuries [21–23]. Ballet dancers who train for more than 5 hours per day have a significantly higher stress fracture risk than those who train for less than 5 hours daily [24].

Abrupt or rapid changes in duration, frequency, or intensity of training programs also increase an athlete's risk of stress fracture. Reducing the intensity or frequency of the training program led to fewer stress fractures in female and male military recruits [25–27]; however, this intervention has not been studied in athletes.

*Footwear.* Athletic footwear is designed to reduce impact on ground contact and provide stability by controlling foot and ankle motion [28]. Shoe age is a better indicator of shock-absorbing quality than shoe cost. Gardner et al [29] showed that training in shoes that are older than 6 months increases the risk for stress fracture; however, there has been no association between shoe cost and stress fracture risk [29]. A woman's foot has a greater forefoot to hindfoot ratio, which can result in poor shoe fit and leave the hindfoot less

---

**Box 2. Risk factors for stress fractures**

*Extrinsic*
Training regimen
Footwear
Training surface
Type of sport

*Intrinsic*
Demographic factors
  Gender
  Age
  Race
  Aerobic fitness
  Muscle strength
  Flexibility
Biomechanical factors
  Bone mineral density
  Bone geometry
Anatomic factors
  Foot morphology
  Leg length discrepancy
  Knee alignment
Hormonal factors
  Delayed menarche
  Menstrual disturbance
  Contraception
Nutritional factors
  Low calcium and vitamin D intake
  Disordered eating

---

supported. Custom made biomechanical shoe orthoses that place the foot in neutral subtalar position and absorb shock decreased the overall incidence of stress fractures in infantry recruits [30,31]; however, this may not be applicable to running athletes [32].

*Training surface.* The surface on which an athlete trains also may contribute to her risk of stress fracture. Theoretically, training on uneven surfaces could increase the risk of stress fracture by causing increased muscle fatigue and redistributing load to bone. Hard or less compliant surfaces, such as cement, also could increase stress fracture risk through higher mechanical forces being transmitted to bone during impact. It is difficult to control for and quantify training surface in observational or prospective studies; however, a correlation was demonstrated in some studies [21,33], whereas others showed no effect [20,23]. One small study found treadmill runners to be at lower risk for developing tibial stress fracture, but also less likely to achieve tibial bone strengthening, than overground runners [33].

*Type of sport.* An Australian study in 1994 quantified the rate of stress fracture in men and women in different sports. In this study, the percentage of athletes per season who had stress fractures were as follows: softball 6.3%, track 3.7%, basketball 2.9%, tennis 2.8%, gymnastics 2.8%, lacrosse 2.7%, baseball 2.6%, volleyball 2.4%, crew 2.2%, and field hockey 2.2% [34]. Sprinters, hurdlers, and jumpers tended to have more foot fractures, whereas middle and long-distance runners had more long bone and pelvic fractures [35]. Rowers and golfers have increased rates of rib stress fractures [36,37].

*Intrinsic risk factors*
*Demographic factors.* Most studies have found that women have a higher incidence of stress fractures. It is probably multifactorial, and secondary, at least in part, to gender-associated risk factors, such as dietary deficiencies, menstrual irregularities, lower BMD, and narrower bone width. Gender differences in muscle physiology, especially neuromuscular control, also may be to blame. Several studies have shown that women have a slower rate of force development in the muscle [38–40].

In the U.S. military, the risk of stress fractures in female recruits who undergo the same training program as men is up to 10 times higher [4]. This increased risk also has been observed in athletic populations [34,41,42]. Bennell et al [35] reported no difference in the overall stress fracture incidence between male and female athletes; however, the data seem to show a trend for a higher risk of stress fractures in women when the amount of training hours were taken into account. Women, however, seem to have more femoral neck, metatarsal, and pelvic stress fractures than men [43]. Further research is needed to determine whether the apparent higher incidence of stress fractures in women is independent of other known risk factors.

The role of age as a risk for stress fractures in female athletes is not established. Studies in military recruits have been inconsistent, with some finding an increased risk of stress fractures with increasing age [44,45] and others finding a decreased risk [29,46–48] or no effect [49,50]. This lack of agreement is most likely due to confounding factors, such as previous physical activity level, hormonal status, BMD, and training level. Most studies in athletic populations have not found a correlation between age and stress fracture risk, although rigorous studies that controlled for other possible confounding variables are lacking.

The incidence of stress fractures is significantly higher in white and Asian women than in African American women [29,44–46]. This is believed to be related to differences in bone turnover and peak bone density and not to race independently. It also seems that ethnic differences in bone mineralization and bone integrity in athletes are mediated by heritable differences in titratable acid, sodium, and calcium excretion [51].

Previously inactive or less active military recruits have a higher incidence of stress fractures compared with those who are active before beginning basic training [29,48,49]. Several possible factors include decreased aerobic fitness, decreased muscle strength, lower endurance, and poor flexibility. A study of military recruits found no association between aerobic fitness (predicted $Vo_2max$) and stress fracture risk [52]. It is unlikely that aerobic fitness alone accounts for the difference [53,54]. The role of flexibility on stress fractures has not been well-defined [35,47,55].

*Biomechanical factors.* Lower BMD, especially of the femoral neck, was associated with an increased risk of stress fractures in the female athlete [56]. Although there are published case-control studies that support [57] and refute [49] this finding, Bennell and colleagues [53] were the first to examine this prospectively. They found that lower BMD in the lumbar spine and foot were significant predictors of later stress fracture development in female track and field athletes. Of note, an athlete with an apparently normal BMD (due to the increased bone loading of sport) may be at increased risk of stress fracture if she falls below the mean among female athletes. It also was observed in athletic females that cancellous stress fractures correlate with early onset osteopenia by Dual Energy Xray Absortiometry scan much more so than cortical bone stress fractures [58]. This indicates the necessity of bone density evaluation in any young woman who has a cancellous stress fracture. Menstrual disturbance and lower BMD most likely are not risk factors that are independent of each other, but are interrelated; amenorrheic athletes have lower BMD and higher stress fracture incidence [59].

The amount of force that a bone can withstand is proportional to its cross-sectional area and cross-sectional moment of inertia (a measure of bone resistance to bending). Studies of military personnel found these parameters to be significantly lower among those who develop stress fractures [60–62]. They also found that of persons who sustained femoral, tibial, or foot stress fractures, 31% had narrowed tibial width compared with those without fracture [63]. This narrowed tibial width may be an indicator of biomechanically weaker skeletal structures. It is hypothesized that women are likely to have overall narrower bones than men [64]; this is a possible contributing factor to the higher incidence of stress fractures in women.

*Anatomic factors.* The structure of the foot helps to determine how much ground contact force is absorbed in the foot and how much is transferred to the bones of the leg and thigh. A rigid, high-arched foot (pes cavus) absorbs less stress and transmits greater force to the tibia and femur. A flexible, low-arched foot (pes planus) absorbs more force in the foot itself and transmits less to the tibia, fibula, and femur. One military study that evaluated foot morphology found that persons who had the highest arches sustained 3.9 times as many stress fractures as those who had the lowest arches [65]. Other studies [65,66] suggest that individuals who have pes cavus seem to be at increased risk of tibial and femoral stress fractures, whereas those who have pes planus may sustain more metatarsal stress fractures. Other investigators have not found a significant correlation between foot structure and stress fracture risk [20,53]. It is possible that pes planus and pes cavus foot structure may increase the risk of stress fracture at various sites, but this has not been evaluated adequately or proven.

Leg length discrepancy also has been associated with an increased risk of stress fractures in female athletes [20,53]. The degree of leg length difference may correlate with increasing stress fracture risk [67]; however, one study of male military recruits did not confirm this relationship [68]. It is reasonable to evaluate and correct significant leg length discrepancy in runners, especially those with other stress fracture risks.

Valgus knee alignment and quadriceps angle greater than 15° also may increase the risk for tibial stress fracture [68,69].

*Hormonal factors.* Female athletes, in general, reach menarche at a later age than nonathletes, particularly those in certain sports, such as ballet, running, and gymnastics [70,71]. Delayed menarche may cause lower peak bone mass attainment or may be a marker for other possible influences on stress fracture risk, such as low body fat, low body weight, future menstrual disturbance, or excessive training. The effect of this delay on bone health and risk of stress fractures is not well-studied; however, some studies suggest that osteopenia, stress fracture, and scoliosis may be potential complications of delayed menarche [53,71]. Scoliosis, in particular, has been observed in female ballet dancers with delayed menarche [71]. This also may lead to pelvic obliquity and relative leg length discrepancies and the potential for increasing the risk for stress fracture.

Multiple studies have demonstrated that stress fractures occur more commonly in women who have amenorrhea or oligomenorrhea than in eumenorrheic women [17,46,48,53,57,71]. Athletes who have menstrual disturbances have low basal estrogen concentrations [72] and a lower BMD than eumenorrheic athletes [73]. It was hypothesized that estrogen deprivation increases the physiologic set point for bone modeling and remodeling and makes it more difficult to activate the cellular response that is necessary to induce bone adaptation to stress [4,74] and increases the risk of stress fractures. Health care providers, athletes, coaches, and parents need to be aware that menstrual disturbance is not a normal product of training and that such disturbances can have devastating consequences. Menstrual disturbances also are seen in association with disordered eating and endothelial cell dysfunction (see "The female athlete Triad," below). Therefore, athletes who have menstrual irregularity should be evaluated further.

Some studies have shown that oral contraceptive pills (OCPs) have a protective effect in preventing stress fractures in female athletes [17,75]. It seems that exogenous estrogen may help to curb further bone loss in the hypoestrogenic amenorrheic athlete; however, it may not be sufficient to stimulate bone growth [71,76–79]. Several small studies among amenorrheic women or those who had anorexia found that BMD at the lumbar spine or hip was higher for those who were taking OCPs compared with those who were not [76,77,80], whereas others showed no significant change [71,78]. It also was theorized that OCPs may act through another mechanism, such as improving bone microarchitecture and quality without significantly affecting BMD [4]. To add to the controversy, a recent German study by Hartard et al [81] showed that OCP use is associated with decreased BMD of the spine (7.9%) and the femoral neck (8.8%) in female endurance athletes compared with non-OCP users. They also found that early age at initiation of OCPs was an important risk factor for low peak bone mass in young women. Based on the conflicting results from research and the lack of well-controlled studies, it is difficult to assess the effects of OCPs on skeletal health in normally menstruating women. In those who have menstrual disturbances, OCPs or other hormonal replacement therapy may be effective in preventing further bone loss; however, resumption of menses may mask an underlying nutritional disorder and provide a false sense of security. Recent evidence also suggests that depomedroxyprogesterone may contribute to impaired bone accretion and low BMD, and it should be avoided in young women [82].

*Nutritional factors.* Low calcium intake is associated with low BMD [83], and therefore, may contribute to the development of stress fractures. Myburgh and colleagues [57] observed an association between decreased calcium intake and increased stress fracture risk. Other studies found no association between calcium intake and stress fracture risk; groups that did and did not have stress fractures had normal calcium intake [13,84,85]. Athletes whose calcium intake is less than the daily-recommended value are likely to be at risk for stress fractures, but for those who have a normal dietary calcium intake, other factors play a larger role.

Vitamin D also is essential to bone health and functions, including stimulating calcium transport, osteoblastic stimulation, and decreasing parathyroid hormone. Recent studies focus on the role of the vitamin D receptor allele in predicting bone density. More research is necessary to determine the clinical applications of its use in screening [86–88].

Inadequate caloric intake relative to energy expenditure that is required for seems to be the primary mechanism by which female athletes are predisposed to menstrual dysfunction and detrimental effects on bone. Anorexia nervosa has been associated with a significantly decreased BMD [7,89]. Nearly 75% of adolescent girls who had anorexia had a BMD that was more than two standard deviations below the normal value [90]. Not surprisingly, women who have anorexia nervosa are at increased risk for stress fracture development [91,92]. Disordered eating is associated with low BMD in the absence of menstrual irregularities [59].

## The female athlete triad

The female athlete triad refers to an interrelated problem that consists of disordered eating, amenorrhea, and osteoporosis. Hoch et al [93] also found that amenorrheic athletes had reduced brachial artery endothelium-dependent flow-mediated vasodilation when compared with oligomenorrheic and eumenorrheic athletes. Furthermore, in a 2-year follow-up study, the original amenorrheic athletes had a significant improvement in BMD with different combinations of estrogen and progesterone or return of menses naturally. This female athlete triad is a potentially lethal combination of medical disorders that is reported in some female athletes [4,42]. Athletes who are at greatest risk seem to be those who feel significant pressure to excel in sports for which leanness and a low body weight are considered advantageous, such as gymnastics, figure skating, ballet, and distance running [94]. Also, athletes who participate in individual sports are at higher risk than those who participate in team sports.

The problem usually begins with disordered eating; this includes a spectrum of abnormal and harmful eating patterns, such as bingeing and purging, restrictive eating, fasting, and the use of diet pills or laxatives. Preoccupation with food, a distorted body image, and intense fear of becoming fat are often present as well. Some athletes will meet the *Diagnostic and Statistical Manual of Mental Disorders, Fourth Edition* criteria for anorexia nervosa or bulimia, whereas others may display similar behaviors without meeting full diagnostic criteria. A new classification—eating disorder, not otherwise specified—allows for identification of women who do not meet other classification criteria. This has been helpful in this population because the athlete's weight may seem to be adequate because of increased lean tissue mass; however, they are not consuming enough calories to meet their energy needs.

Abnormal eating patterns may lead to athletic-associated amenorrhea. Athletic amenorrhea is a complex multifactorial condition with serious associated comorbidities. Extreme caloric restriction, excessive exercise, physical and emotional stress that are associated with exercise/competition, percentage of body fat, and genetics contribute to the condition. There is increasing evidence, however, that nutritional restrictions and the resulting endocrine and metabolic changes are a critical initiator of hypothalamic-induced athletic amenorrhea and osteoporosis [95].

Disordered eating, estrogen deficiency, and menstrual dysfunction predispose women to the third component of the triad, osteoporosis [89]. Reduced BMD in premenopausal women seems to be irreversible, despite weight gain, resumption of menses, or estrogen replacement [6,7]. One study found that with the resumption of menses there was a significant increase in vertebral BMD; however, after 2 years of normal menses, BMD remained below age-normative. Slemenda et al [96] showed that the low estrogenic state that is associated with amenorrhea has a more profound effect on cancellous bone than on cortical bone. Cancellous bone is found in a higher percentage in the pelvis, sacrum, and femoral neck—areas where females tend to have a higher occurrence of stress fractures. These factors put the woman who suffers from the female athlete triad at significant risk for stress fractures. Although some investigators found that weight-bearing exercise has a skeletal protective effect and may attenuate the bone loss that usually is seen in anorexics [89], the use of excessive training to control weight also could contribute to the increased risk of stress fractures that is associated with the female athlete triad.

Several other factors are known to increase the risk for osteoporosis but have not been investigated thoroughly as possible risks for stress fractures in female athletes. These include smoking, caffeine consumption, and certain medications, such as thyroid hormone and corticosteroids. In a study of female army recruits, current or past smoking, consumption of more than 10 alcoholic drinks/week, corticosteroid use, use of depomedroxyprogesterone acetate, lower adult weight, and no history of regular exercise increased the likelihood of stress fracture [45,82].

## Screening and prevention of stress injury in female runners

Ideally, stress fractures and the female athlete triad are treated best through prevention. With many of the risk factors for stress fracture now known, screening and prevention are much easier. Evaluation of all components of the triad should be performed on every female runner. A thorough history is essential and should include assessments of nutrition; amount of, and changes in, physical activity; and menstrual history. A history of stress fractures or overuse injuries as well as signs or symptoms of an eating disorder justify further evaluation. Characteristics of anorexia nervosa include cachexia, bradycardia, hypotension, lanugo, hypothermia, cold intolerance, yellow skin (hypercarotenemia), dry hair and skin, alopecia, and pruritus. Signs and symptoms of bulimia include fatigue, abdominal pain, chest pain, swollen parotid glands, sore throat, eroded tooth enamel, and knuckle calluses. Screening with bone density testing should be considered in athletes who have known risk factors. The diagnosis of osteoporosis in premenopausal women should not be made on the basis of densitometric criteria alone. It also is not appropriate to use T-scores when peak bone mass has not been reached; therefore, athletes who are 20 years old and younger should be evaluated with Z-scores [97]. Treatment of the triad often requires a team approach. A sports physician, dietitian, and psychologist may be needed to work with the athlete in addition to her coach, parents, and close friends. Treatment for underlying disordered eating, correction of an energy deficit, and restoration of menses are essential to stimulate bone accretion. Nutritional supplementation with calcium and vitamin D and reduced training may be recommended. Early intervention speeds recovery.

Reductions in bone density and an increased risk of stress fracture are noted when there is an uncoupling of bone formation and resorption rates as seen when energy availability is too low [59]. Several metabolic hormones that influence bone formation (IGF-1, $T_3$, leptin), as well as bone formation markers (serum type I procollagen carboxyl-terminal propeptide, osteocalcin) and bone resorption markers (urine N-telopeptide, serum C-telopeptide), can be followed to form an impression of the overall bone turnover status and assess energy status indirectly. Uncoupling of bone resorption and formation is seen with restricted energy availability as little as 126 kJ/kg of lean body mass/d [12]. Therefore, increasing caloric intake to offset the high energy demand may help to restore menses and stimulate bone accretion. Calcium intakes of 1200 mg/d to 1500 mg/d and 400 IU to 800 IU of vitamin D also help to minimize bone loss. Antiresorptive therapies, such as bisphosphonates and calcitonin, have not been tested and are not approved by the U.S. Food and Drug Administration in younger patients who have reduced BMD/osteoporosis. Their use in this population is controversial; they are teratogenic and have a half-life in bone of greater than 10 years.

Treatment with exogenous estrogens has been evaluated in numerous studies with varying results. It seems that this may help to reduce further bone loss in hypoestrogenic amenorrheic athletes; however, it may be insufficient to stimulate bone growth [79]. Another concern is that with the restoration of menses, estrogen replacement may mask the underlying disorder. Recent evidence suggests that depomedroxyprogesterone acetate contributes to impaired bone accretion and loss in mean BMD and should be avoided in amenorrheic athletes [82]. Other preventative measures include not smoking and the minimal use of alcohol [45].

Because training errors frequently are the cause of stress fractures, any abrupt increase in training should be avoided. Cyclical training—a limited period of training followed by relative rest during the third week (the interval of greatest skeletal vulnerability)—is recommended over progressive training [25]. For runners, mileage increases should be gradual, with some investigators recommending that mileage should not be increased by more than 3.2 total km/wk [98]. Using shock-absorbing insoles and changing shoes every 6 months or before 800 km also is recommended.

*Diagnosis of stress fractures*

The treatment of stress fractures starts with a specific and accurate diagnosis. Diagnosis of stress fractures often can be difficult and requires a high degree of suspicion. A thorough history and physical examination often diagnoses most stress fractures successfully. The onset of pain with an abrupt change in training, such as increasing mileage or intensity, should raise suspicion of a stress fracture. Pain typically occurs at the end of, or after, a run. Point tenderness on physical examination is the hallmark. For example, the so-called "N-spot" on the dorsum of the navicular can be a site of exquisite tenderness in runners who have navicular stress fractures. Swelling and redness may be present, but deformity usually is not. Percussion tapping of bone, vibrating tuning fork, single leg hop, femoral fulcrum, and lumbar extension tests (for pars stress fracture) are nonspecific physical examination maneuvers that help in the identification of stress fractures. Application of stress to the area or passive stretching also can reproduce pain [99]. If multiple or recurrent stress fractures are present, evaluation for sources of metabolic bone disease and the female athlete triad is warranted. Some stress fractures are considered to be at high risk (Box 3) for nonunion and should be treated aggressively, often with a period of nonweight bearing, and perhaps, surgery [106]. These high-risk fractures include ones at the femoral neck, the mid shaft of the tibia, and the navicular.

The most common location of stress fractures in runners is the tibia; however, tibial stress fractures may be difficult to discern from so-called "shin splints," more properly termed medial tibial stress syndrome (MTSS). Typically, pain with stress fractures worsens as the run goes on. Occasionally with MTSS, pain may diminish as the runner warms up. Physical examination reveals focal tenderness with tibial stress fractures, whereas MTSS presents with diffuse tenderness (with maximal tenderness at the junction between the middle and distal third of the medial tibia). Percussion tenderness, a tuning fork test, or hop tests are more likely to be

---

**Box 3. High-risk stress fractures that require aggressive treatment**

Femoral neck
Anterior cortex or midshaft of tibia
Navicular
Medial malleolus
Talus fracture extending to subtalar joint
Proximal second metatarsal
Proximal fifth metatarsal diaphysis (Jones fracture)
Sesamoid
Pars interarticularis

---

*Data from* Fredericson M, Bergman AG, Matheson GO. [Stress fractures in athletes] [German]. Orthopade 1997;26(11):961.

positive with tibial stress fractures than with MTSS. Posterior cortex tibial stress fractures can present with calf pain rather than shin pain.

A definitive diagnosis of a stress fracture often requires imaging. Plain radiographs have poor sensitivity but are highly specific and are recommended as an initial step in diagnosis. The "gray cortex" sign may be evident on the radiograph if the cortex has decreased density with associated hyperemia, edema, and early resorption [106]. The "dreaded black line" also can be seen on radiograph in individuals who have a midshaft tibia fracture that has failed to heal and developed a nonunion [106]. Many of these will be falsely negative as callus formation can take up to 3 months to appear. If suspicion is high with negative radiographs, conservative treatment should be initiated followed by repeat evaluation and radiographs in 2 weeks. If the injury is in the season of competition, it is reasonable to perform further imaging before implementing the 2-week rest.

MRI and bone scintigraphy (triple phase bone scan) have comparable sensitivity and either is acceptable. MRI is preferred because it is less invasive; avoids radiation exposure (an important consideration in this young female population); has better specificity (ie, can differentiate fracture from tumor); and shows more diagnostic information, such as fracture line and periosteal edema. MRI can show stress changes, or edema, within the bone, even before a fracture develops. Fat-suppressed T2-weighted images also are recommended to help identify any bone marrow edema. Areas of increased activity by scintigraphy seem to be consistent with grades of MRI [99,100]. The main drawback of MRI, aside from cost, is that it does not image cortical bone as well as CT. CT is useful in differentiating conditions that may mimic stress fracture on bone scan, such as osteoid osteoma, osteomyelitis with Brodie's abscess, and various malignancies. It is also helpful in detecting fracture lines as evidence of stress fractures and often can differentiate between stress fracture and stress reaction [101]. This is particularly important in the elite athlete as it may affect their rehabilitation program and upcoming competitions considerably. Ultrasound is not reliable in diagnosing stress fractures and is not recommended [102].

*Conservative treatment for stress fractures*

Conservative treatment for stress fractures is a three-part protocol using pain as a guide to rehabilitation. Phase 1 includes cessation of painful activity, ice, analgesics, maintaining fitness by cross-training, modification of risk factors, and possible bracing or electrical stimulation [101]. It is important that the runner who has a stress fracture be able to maintain aerobic fitness and strength during the healing period. The most common ways to unweight the fractured extremity and maintain cardiovascular fitness are cycling, water running, and swimming. Cross-training should be as sport specific as possible in duration and intensity. Extrinsic factors, especially training errors, need to be addressed because these are the most common cause of stress fractures. Particularly important to female runners are intrinsic conditions, such as disordered eating, amenorrhea, and premature osteoporosis. Moreover, certain stress fractures occur in areas of hypovascularity and are at risk for nonunion or avascular necrosis; in these cases, surgery should be considered.

Adjunctive therapies, such as pneumatic braces or capacitative coupling, also may be instituted. The use of pneumatic braces in the rehabilitation of tibial stress fractures seems to reduce the time to recommencing training in athletes and military personnel; it allowed resumption of light activity in 7 days (median) and full, unrestricted activity in 21 ± 2 days versus 21 days (median) and 77 ± 7 days with rest alone [31,103]. Capacitative coupling also has been used to shorten healing time. Stress fractures typically take 8 to 12 weeks to heal; however, one study found that healing time with capacitative coupling was shortened to 7 weeks on average [104]. Weight-bearing trials should be performed every other day. After 3 to 5 days free from pain, phase 2 begins.

Phase 2 consists of light-weighted exercises and nonimpact-loading activities, such as walking, using a stair stepper, elliptical, or cross-country skiing machine. Activity should resume slowly and increase by 5 to 10 minutes per day up to 45 minutes. If any bony pain occurs, activity should stop for 1 to 2 days and restart at a level below which the pain occurred [101,105]. Recovery of strength that is lost during phase 1 also should be addressed. Sport-specific muscle rehabilitation also may be started.

Phase 3 is gradual re-entry into the athlete's sport-specific activity, starting every other day and gradually progressing to normal activity. This program may take from 3 to 18 weeks, depending on the extent of the injury [105]. All athletes also should have a biomechanical and gait evaluation to assess for leg length abnormalities, excessive pronation or supination, pes planus, pes cavus, and other structural abnormalities following a stress fracture.

## Knee injuries

The knee joint is an innocent bystander in the lower limb kinetic chain (ie, injuries at the knee usually are the result of biomechanical problems above or below the knee). The differential diagnosis of knee pain in the runner is described in Table 1.

### Patellofemoral pain syndrome

Patellofemoral pain syndrome (PFPS) is the most common diagnosis for knee pain in athletic and nonathletic populations; the incidence may be twice as high in female athletes compared with their male counterparts [107,108]. Adolescent females seem to be at particular risk because their accelerated bony changes have not been accommodated by muscle changes

Table 1
Differential diagnosis of knee pain

| Medial | Lateral | Anterior | Posterior |
| --- | --- | --- | --- |
| PFPS | PFPS | PFPS | Baker's cyst |
| Plica | ITBS | Quadriceps tend. | Hamstring tend. |
| MMT | Popliteus | Patellar tend. | Popliteus |
| MCL sprain | LCL sprain | Patellar instability | |
| Intra-articular | LMT | Hoffa's syndrome | |
| Osteoarthritis | Intra-articular | Patellar OCD | |
| MMT | Osteoarthritis | Osteoarthritis | |
| | | Bursitis | |

*Abbreviations:* ITBS, iliotibial band syndrome; LCL, lateral collateral ligament; LMT, lateral meniscus tear; MCL, medical collateral ligament; MMT, medical meniscus tear; OCD, osteochondral defect; PFPS, patellofemoral pain syndrome; tend., tendinopathy.

[107]. The PFPS pain syndrome is an amalgam of diagnoses and generally can be classified into patellar instability, PFPS with malalignment, and PFPS without malalignment.

*Patellofemoral pain syndrome pain generators*

Traditional thinking has assumed that the patellar cartilage is the primary pain generator in the PFPS. Accordingly, the term "chondromalacia patellae" often is used for nebulous anterior knee pain; however, there are no nerve endings in the articular cartilage [109]. Arthroscopy studies also have failed to correlate the degree of patellar chondral and subchondral injury with the severity of anterior knee pain [109]. The current theory of pathogenesis is injury to the subchondral bone from patellar maltracking and increased patellofemoral joint reaction forces. Dye et al [110] proposed that the actual pain generator is the loading of nerve endings (ie, a degenerative neuroma) in the patellar retinaculum which causes a resultant synovitis. Other pain generators may exist in PFPS, such as irritated infrapatellar fat pad, plica, bursa, tendons, and apophyses.

*Predisposing factors for patellofemoral pain syndrome*

Biomechanical structural problems may contribute to patellofemoral pain [109]. For instance, miserable malalignment syndrome in women predisposes to PFPS. Muscle imbalances may exacerbate knee pain. Weak quadriceps musculature, particularly the vastus medialis obliquis (VMO) portion, has been implicated in patellofemoral pain. When the VMO is weak or inhibited, lateral vector forces that are created by the vastus lateralis, iliotibial band (ITB), and lateral retinaculum become dominant. Thus, the patella becomes displaced laterally. Tight lateral structures (ITB and lateral retinaculum) exacerbate this phenomena. Specifically in runners, a tight ITB and tensor fascia lata muscle, coupled with weak gluteus medius, creates excessive internal rotation of the femur and a lateral pelvic tilt. Tight hamstrings and gastrocnemius musculature also may exacerbate PFPS by increasing knee flexion and creating greater patellofemoral joint reaction forces. In addition, hyperpronation seems to predispose runners to PFPS.

*Clinical presentation*

The classic presentation of PFPS is an insidious onset of progressively severe diffuse anterior knee pain, especially with loading activities that involve repetitive flexion and extension, such as running. It may manifest as an ill-defined, usually bilateral, ache which is aggravated by hill training or stair climbing. Knee buckling can occur occasionally as a result of a painful reflex inhibition of the knee extensor mechanism. Other complaints may include crepitus or a "catching" sensation that is experienced with knee joint flexion and extension; however, crepitus may be common, even in asymptomatic individuals. Prolonged sitting with knee flexion, such as on an airplane flight or in a theater, may aggravate patellofemoral pain and lead individuals to extend their knee and legs into the aisle, also known as the "movie theater sign."

In runners, patellar or quadriceps tendinopathy can occur, which is manifested as pinpoint pain at the inferior and superior pole of the patella, respectively. Occasionally, patellar instability symptoms can occur with descriptions of the "knee cap slipping out." Infrapatellar fat pad impingement, occurs with forceful knee extension in individuals who have a prominent fat pad and posterior tilting of the patella. In adolescent runners, apophysitis of the inferior pole of the patella (Sinding-Larsen-Johansen syndrome) or at the tibial tuberosity (Osgood-Schlatter syndrome) should be suspected [111].

*Diagnosis*

The history and physical evaluation of the runner who has knee pain should include analysis of the kinetic chain. Plain radiographs, particularly lateral and "sunrise" (or "skyline") views, may be helpful in evaluating the patellofemoral joint [112]. Sunrise radiographs are axial views that are taken with the knee flexed 30° or 45°. If the patellofemoral joints shows joint space narrowing, osteophytes, subchondral sclerosis, and cysts, patellofemoral osteoarthritis should be suspected. Osteochondral lesions sometimes can be seen with these views. The lateral radiograph may demonstrate patella alta, rotational malalignment, or trochlear dysplasia. More commonly, particularly in the younger female runner who has PFPS, these radiographs are normal. Occasionally, MRI is useful in identifying the quality of the patellar cartilage pathology and ruling out other knee pathologies.

*Treatment*

In general, the management for PFPS should be individualized and aimed at symptom relief acutely, and then focus on correcting the etiologic factors that contribute to the pain. The patient should be reminded that successful alleviation and prevention of further discomfort with PFPS might take several weeks to months. In the authors' experience, patellar tendinopathy cases may take even longer with a longer period of relative unloading.

*Acute phase.* Relative rest is often helpful in alleviating patellofemoral pain. Runners often benefit from switching to low-impact aerobic activities for a defined period of time, such as swimming, aqua aerobics, "elliptical" training, or biking. Biking may exacerbate PFPS if the seat is too high or too low or if increased resistance is maintained. Runners who have PFPS should avoid step aerobics or using the stair-climbing apparatus because these can cause tremendous repetitive compressive loads on the patellofemoral joint. Patellar tendinopathy cases often need 2 to 3 weeks of relative unloading of the tendon.

In the acutely swollen knee, ice may provide some relief from the acute discomfort. Although anti-inflammatory medications have not been shown conclusively to benefit chronic PFPS, nonsteroidal anti-inflammatory drugs or acetaminophen may have a role in acute pain. Glucosamine/chondroitin also has been suggested to provide relief in PFPS, particularly if osteo-arthritis is demonstrated on imaging [113].

*Rehabilitation phase.* Physical therapy was shown to be efficacious in relieving pain in PFS in uncontrolled, and, more recently, controlled trials [114]. Crossley et al's [114] program outlines elements of physical therapy intervention that can be used on all individuals (Box 4). It stands to reason that a more individualized program that attacks specific biomechanical deficits may be even more effective. Closed kinetic chain exercises serve as the cornerstone of the muscle strengthening program in PFPS. Studies showed that although open and closed kinetic chain exercises seem to improve PFPS symptoms, closed chain exercises also seem to improve functional performance. In particular, the literature has emphasized VMO strengthening in the open and closed kinetic chain positions [109]. Isokinetic open chain exercises also have been used for lower limb strengthening; however, they require specialized equipment and are not functional. For patients who are in acute pain, isometric exercises may be painless and just as beneficial as isokinetic exercise. A stretching program, as outlined by Crossley et al [114], also has a sound theoretic basis in eliminating biomechanical deficits.

Debate exists about whether VMO strengthening is important and whether VMO can be strengthened preferentially [115,116]. Some studies suggest that VMO firing is delayed in patients who have patellofemoral pain [115]; however, a robust relationship has yet to be established. A recent study revealed that nine common exercises that are given for preferential VMO strengthening showed equal firing of all of the different portions of the quadriceps [117]. Based on that study, some investigators have advocated for a generalized quadriceps strengthening program, rather than a selective VMO strengthening program. Other researchers showed that patients who

---

**Box 4. Elements of physical therapy intervention**

*Stretches*
  Medial/lateral glides and mobilization of the patella
  Deep friction massage to lateral soft tissues
  Hamstring stretch
  Anterior hip stretch
*Patellar taping*
*Strengthening*
  Isometric VMO strengthening with knees at 90°
  Partial squats with isometric gluteal contraction
  Isometric hip abduction against wall while standing
  Step-downs with pelvis parallel to floor
  Isometric hip abduction while standing away from wall
  Lunges
*Home exercise program: two times per day*
*Surface EMG*

---

*Adapted from* Crossley K, Bennell K, Green S, Cowan S, McConnell J. Physical therapy for patellofemoral pain. Am J Sports Med 2002;30(6):860.

---

have PFPS can learn the motor skill of selectively firing the VMO with patellar taping or EMG biofeedback [118,119]. These patients may have a better short-term outcome [119].

*Patellar taping, braces, and foot orthoses.* Some investigators believe that taping the patella may improve patellar alignment, tracking, tilt, or glide. Although numerous studies have been performed on this intervention for the treatment of PFPS, there are variable results [109,113,120]; however, in the authors' clinical practice, runners who perform a single leg squat and have improvement of pain with manual force on the patella may benefit from patellar taping. Patellar taping is continued only if a 50% reduction of pain is achieved [120]. Patellar taping likely works by reducing pain and improving proprioception rather than by way of a true improvement of patellar orientation. Taping may be especially beneficial in infrapatellar pad impingement by unloading the inflamed fat pad.

Elastic knee sleeves that have an anterior cut-out over the patella may provide some comfort, and because of their low cost, may be a useful strategy in some cases; however, the ability of the sleeve to alter patellar biomechanics is not known, and if used, should be an adjunct with therapeutic exercises. More expensive, more elaborate knee braces have not been shown to be particularly effective in patients who have PFPS [121].

Foot orthoses have been theorized to improve the biomechanics in the lower extremity, including the improvement of patellar tracking [122]. In a study of 20 adolescent girls who had PFPS and exhibited excessive forefoot varus or hindfoot valgus, individuals who were treated with foot orthoses and an exercise regimen had a significant decrease in the level of pain over an 8-week period compared with the control group who underwent exercises alone [123]. It is more economical to try off-the-shelf orthoses first to determine whether the patient derives any benefit initially, and progress to custom orthoses if increased support is required.

*Surgery.* Nonsurgical options in the treatment plan for PFPS should be attempted first; however, more than 100 surgical options have been described for persistent patellofemoral pain that is nonresponsive to conservative treatment. Lateral retinacular release may be the most common procedure that is performed. It works best in individuals who have isolated lateral patellar tilt as the primary cause of patellar malalignment. Lateral retinacular release does not correct a more global malpositioning of the patella nor a large dynamic Q-angle. Inappropriate lateral release can lead to medial patellar subluxation, which can be a debilitating problem. Other more extensive realignment procedures can be performed experimentally to correct Q-angles and patellar orientation. These procedures typically do not allow athletes to return to running activity [120].

Articular cartilage procedures may include open or arthroscopically-performed debridement or shaving of patellar cartilage to achieve a smoother patellofemoral articulation, local excision of defects with drilling of the subchondral bone, or facetectomy and transplantation of autologous chondrocytes [124]. Local excision of diseased cartilage and subchondral drilling has been used commonly with satisfactory results, especially in patients who are younger than 25 years [124]. The long-term results of these articular cartilage procedures are not known, and the relative effectiveness of one procedure compared with the others also is unknown. Their role, although commonplace, is still experimental.

## Iliotibial band friction syndrome

In runners, the next most common knee injury is ITB friction syndrome (ITBS). The ITB is dense fascia that connects the gluteal muscles to the anterolateral tibia. An anatomic pouch can be found underlying the posterior ITB at the level of the lateral femoral epicondyle. The ITB passes over the lateral femoral epicondyle with knee flexion and extension. Maximum friction occurs when the posterior fibers of the ITB pass over the lateral femoral epicondyle at 20° to 30° of knee flexion—the putative "impingement zone." Repeated knee flexion and extension, particularly with increased mileage per week, was shown to predispose to lateral knee pain. Although not studied extensively, poor neuromuscular control seems to be an important modifiable risk factor for ITBS. Specifically, the neuromuscular system is needed to control the valgus/internal rotation vectors at the knee after heel strike. If appropriate control is not available, the ITB may have an abrupt increase in tension at its insertion site. Strengthening the gluteus medius and tensor fascia lata, which are decelerators of the valgus/internal rotation vectors at the knee, was shown to ameliorate ITBS.

## Clinical presentation

Symptoms of ITBS can emanate at three typical sites—proximal lateral hip, over the lateral femoral epicondyle, or at Gerdy's tubercle. Runners often note more pain with downhill running because of the increased time that is spent in the impingement zone. Paradoxically, runners state that faster running and sprinting often does not produce pain. Fast running allows the athlete to spend more time in knee angles that are greater than 30°.

## Physical examination

The modified Thomas and Ober tests are used to assess flexibility of the ITB and its attached muscles. Knee tenderness is noted at the lateral femoral epicondyle (above the lateral joint line) or at Gerdy's tubercle. Pain also can be elicited frequently by the Noble compression test which is performed in nonweight-bearing and standing positions; the knee is flexed and extended through the impingement zone (20°–30° of knee flexion) while the examiner applies pressure over the lateral femoral epicondyle.

## Rehabilitation

Successful treatment of ITBS can be achieved by incorporating a comprehensive, kinetic chain–oriented approach. Rehabilitation includes proper stretching of the ITB and associated muscles. A standing ITB stretch with the affected leg crossed over, lateral trunk side-bending to the unaffected side, and overhead arm extension to the unaffected side may be the most effective stretch [125] (Fig. 1). Some muscle groups do not respond to stretch unless myofascial and joint restrictions are addressed concomitantly. A qualified physical therapist or massage therapist can release trigger points and fascial adhesions that are identified on physical examination. Strengthening of weak or inhibited muscles can be started in conjunction with a flexibility program [126]. Weak hip abductors are seen often in patients who have ITBS. Hip abductor strengthening, with single leg squats and step-downs, is an efficacious treatment for runners who have ITBS [127]. The core strengthening concepts that were described previously play an empiric role in prevention and rehabilitation. The final stages of rehabilitation focus on sports-specific activity. Correction of form flaws can be invaluable to a runner. Frequently, runners have form deviations that lead to a *sine qua non* of uncontrolled valgus/internal rotation of the knee.

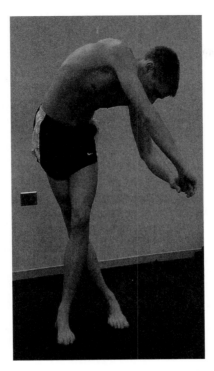

Fig. 1. An effective iliotibial band stretch.

Common abnormalities include excessive pronation, inability to shock attenuate at the knee, and Trendelenburg frontal plane gait at the pelvis. Changing to shock-absorbing or motion-control shoes can accommodate supination and overpronation, respectively. Occasionally, foot orthoses may be helpful in runners who have foot types that exacerbate ITBS.

*Injections and surgery*

Injections that are directed to the anatomic pouch underneath the ITB at the lateral femoral epicondyle is a simple procedure that is used for patients who have persistent pain and swelling. A mixture of anesthetic (eg, 1 mL of 1% lidocaine) and long-acting steroid (eg, 1 mL of betamethasone) is instilled to the affected site [126]. Surgical treatment for ITBS rarely is needed. Surgery involves excising the posterior half of the ITB where it passes over the lateral femoral epicondyle or removing the underlying putative bursa. These surgical procedures give mixed results and should be contemplated only for patients in whom all other options have been exhausted, including a comprehensive rehabilitation program as outlined above.

## Summary

Running often can cause injuries to the knee as a result of kinetic chain dysfunctions. Addressing these dysfunctions in rehabilitation can prevent future injury. Stress fractures often occur in runners who engage in training errors. Female runners are particularly susceptible to stress fractures, especially in the setting of the female athlete triad. Proper identification and prevention of these injuries allows for athletes to return to running expeditiously.

## References

[1] Kaplan FS, Hayes WC, Keaveny TM, et al. Form and function of bone. In: Simon SR, editor. Orthopaedic basic science. Rosemont (IL): American Academy of Orthopaedic Surgeons; 1994. p. 127–94.

[2] Monteleone GP Jr. Stress fractures in the athlete. Orthop Clin N Am 1995;26(3):423–32.

[3] Markey KL. Stress fractures. Clin Sports Med 1987;6(2):405–25.

[4] Nattiv A, Armsey TD Jr. Stress injury to bone in the female athlete. Clin Sports Med 1997; 16(2):197–224.

[5] Theintz G, Buchs B, Rizzoli R, et al. Longitudinal monitoring of bone mass accumulation in healthy adolescents: evidence for a marked reduction after 16 years of age at the levels of lumbar spine and femoral neck in female subjects. J Clin Endocrinol Metab 1992;75(4): 1060–5.

[6] Drinkwater BL, Nilson K, Ott S, et al. Bone mineral density after resumption of menses in amenorrheic athletes. JAMA 1986;256(3):380–2.

[7] Rigotti NA, Neer RM, Skates SJ, et al. The clinical course of osteoporosis in anorexia nervosa. A longitudinal study of cortical bone mass. JAMA 1991;265(9):1133–8.

[8] Zanker CL, Swaine IL. Relation between bone turnover, estradiol, and energy balance in women distance runners. Br J Sports Med 1998;32(2):167–71.

[9] Zanker CL, Swaine IL. Responses of bone turnover markers to repeated endurance running in humans under conditions of energy balance or energy restriction. Eur J Appl Physiol 2000;83(4–5):434–40.

[10] Ammann P, Rizzoli R, Muller K, et al. IGF-I and pamidronate increase bone mineral density in ovariectomized adult rats. Am J Physiol 1993;265(5 Pt 1):E770–6.

[11] Chevalley T, Rizzoli R, Manen D, et al. Arginine increases insulin-like growth factor-I production and collagen synthesis in osteoblast-like cells. Bone 1998;23(2):103–9.

[12] Ihle R, Loucks AB. Dose-response relationships between energy availability and bone turnover in young exercising women. J Bone Miner Res 2004;19(8):1231–40.

[13] Carter DR, Caler WE. A cumulative damage model for bone fracture. J Orthop Res 1985; 3(1):84–90.

[14] Carter DR, Hayes WC. Compact bone fatigue damage: a microscopic examination. Clin Orthop 1977;127:265–74.

[15] Fyhrie DP, Milgrom C, Hoshaw SJ, et al. Effect of fatiguing exercise on longitudinal bone strain as related to stress fracture in humans. Ann Biomed Eng 1998;26(4):660–5.

[16] Otter MW, Qin YX, Rubin CT, et al. Does bone perfusion/reperfusion initiate bone remodeling and the stress fracture syndrome? Med Hypotheses 1999;53(5):363–8.

[17] Barrow GW, Saha S. Menstrual irregularity and stress fractures in collegiate female distance runners. Am J Sports Med 1988;16(3):209–16.

[18] Egol KA, Koval KJ, Kummer F, et al. Stress fractures of the femoral neck. Clin Orthop 1998;348:72–8.

[19] Stanitski CL, McMaster JH, Scranton PE. On the nature of stress fractures. Am J Sports Med 1978;6(6):391–6.
[20] Brunet ME, Cook SD, Brinker MR, et al. A survey of running injuries in 1505 competitive and recreational runners. J Sports Med Phys Fitness 1990;30(3):307–15.
[21] Macera CA, Pate RR, Powell KE, et al. Predicting lower-extremity injuries among habitual runners. Arch Intern Med 1989;149(11):2565–8.
[22] Marti B, Vader JP, Minder CE, et al. On the epidemiology of running injuries. The 1984 Bern Grand-Prix Study. Am J Sports Med 1988;16(3):285–94.
[23] Walter SD, Hart LE, McIntosh JM, et al. The Ontario Cohort Study of Running-Related Injuries. Arch Intern Med 1989;149(11):2561–4.
[24] Kadel NJ, Teitz CC, Kronmal RA. Stress fractures in ballet dancers. Am J Sports Med 1992;20(4):445–9.
[25] Scully TJ, Besterman G. Stress fracture—a preventable training injury. Mil Med 1982; 147(4):285–7.
[26] Rudzki SJ. Injuries in Australian Army recruits. Part I: decreased incidence and severity of injury seen with reduced running distance. Mil Med 1997;162(7):472–6.
[27] Popovich RM, Gardner JW, Potter R, et al. Effect of rest from running on overuse injuries in army basic training. Am J Prev Med 2000;18(3 Suppl):147–55.
[28] Frey C. Footwear and stress fractures. Clin Sports Med 1997;16(2):249–57.
[29] Gardner LI Jr, Dziados JE, Jones BH, et al. Prevention of lower extremity stress fractures: a controlled trial of a shock absorbent insole. Am J Public Health 1988;78(12): 1563–7.
[30] Finestone A, Giladi M, Elad H, et al. Prevention of stress fractures using custom biomechanical shoe orthoses. Clin Orthop 1999;360:182–90.
[31] Gillespie WJ, Grant I. Interventions for preventing and treating stress fractures and stress reactions of bone of the lower limbs in young adults (Cochrane Review). The Cochrane Library, edition 4. Chichester (UK): John Wiley & Sons, LTD; 2004.
[32] Ekenman I, Milgrom C, Finestone A, et al. The role of biomechanical shoe orthoses in tibial stress fracture prevention. Am J Sports Med 2002;30(6):866–70.
[33] Milgrom C, Finestone A, Segev S, et al. Are overground or treadmill runners more likely to sustain tibial stress fracture? Br J Sports Med 2003;37(2):160–3.
[34] Goldberg B, Pecora C. Stress fractures: a risk of increased training in freshman. Phys Sportsmed 1994;22(3):68–78.
[35] Bennell KL, Malcolm SA, Thomas SA, et al. The incidence and distribution of stress fractures in competitive track and field athletes. A twelve-month prospective study. Am J Sports Med 1996;24(2):211–7.
[36] Lord MJ, Ha KI, Song KS. Stress fractures of the ribs in golfers. Am J Sports Med 1996; 24(1):118–22.
[37] Hickey GJ, Fricker PA, McDonald WA. Injuries to elite rowers over a 10-yr period. Med Sci Sports Exerc 1997;29(12):1567–72.
[38] Bell DG, Jacobs I. Electro-mechanical response times and rate of force development in males and females. Med Sci Sports Exerc 1986;18(1):31–6.
[39] Hakkinen K. Force production characteristics of leg extensor, trunk flexor and extensor muscles in male and female basketball players. J Sports Med Phys Fitness 1991;31(3): 325–31.
[40] Winter EM, Brookes FB. Electromechanical response times and muscle elasticity in men and women. Eur J Appl Physiol Occup Physiol 1991;63(2):124–8.
[41] Johnson AW, Weiss CB Jr, Wheeler DL. Stress fractures of the femoral shaft in athletes—more common than expected. A new clinical test. Am J Sports Med 1994;22(2):248–56.
[42] Zernicke RF, McNitt-Gray J, Otis C, et al. Stress fracture risk assessment among elite collegiate women runners. J Biomech 1994;27:854.
[43] Lombardo SJ, Benson DW. Stress fractures of the femur in runners. Am J Sports Med 1982; 10(4):219–27.

[44] Brudvig TJ, Gudger TD, Obermeyer L. Stress fractures in 295 trainees: a one-year study of incidence as related to age, sex, and race. Mil Med 1983;148(8):666–7.

[45] Lappe JM, Stegman MR, Recker RR. The impact of lifestyle factors on stress fractures in female Army recruits. Osteoporos Int 2001;12(1):35–42.

[46] Friedl KE, Nuovo JA, Patience TH, et al. Factors associated with stress fracture in young army women: indications for further research. Mil Med 1992;157(7):334–8.

[47] Milgrom C, Finestone A, Shlamkovitch N, et al. Youth is a risk factor for stress fracture. A study of 783 infantry recruits. J Bone Joint Surg Br 1994;76(1):20–2.

[48] Winfield AC, Moore J, Bracker M, et al. Risk factors associated with stress reactions in female Marines. Mil Med 1997;162(10):698–702.

[49] Cline AD, Jansen GR, Melby CL. Stress fractures in female army recruits: implications of bone density, calcium intake, and exercise. J Am Coll Nutr 1998;17(2):128–35.

[50] Reinker KA, Ozburne S. A comparison of male and female orthopaedic pathology in basic training. Mil Med 1979;144(8):532–6.

[51] Vaitkevicius H, Witt R, Maasdam M, et al. Ethnic differences in titratable acid excretion and bone mineralization. Med Sci Sports Exerc 2002;34(2):295–302.

[52] Swissa A, Milgrom C, Giladi M, et al. The effect of pretraining sports activity on the incidence of stress fractures among military recruits. A prospective study. Clin Orthop 1989;(245):256–60.

[53] Bennell KL, Malcolm SA, Thomas SA, et al. Risk factors for stress fractures in track and field athletes. A twelve-month prospective study. Am J Sports Med 1996;24(6):810–8.

[54] Beck TJ, Ruff CB, Shaffer RA, et al. Stress fracture in military recruits: gender differences in muscle and bone susceptibility factors. Bone 2000;27(3):437–44.

[55] Giladi M, Milgrom C, Stein M, et al. External rotation of the hip. A predictor of risk for stress fractures. Clin Orthop 1987;(216):131–4.

[56] Lauder TD, Dixit S, Pezzin LE, et al. The relation between stress fractures and bone mineral density: evidence from active-duty Army women. Arch Phys Med Rehabil 2000;81(1):73–9.

[57] Myburgh KH, Hutchins J, Fataar AB, et al. Low bone density is an etiologic factor for stress fractures in athletes. Ann Intern Med 1990;113(10):754–9.

[58] Marx RG, Saint-Phard D, Callahan LR, et al. Stress fracture sites related to underlying bone health in athletic females. Clin J Sport Med 2001;11(2):73–6.

[59] Cobb KL, Bachrach LK, Greendale G, et al. Disordered eating, menstrual irregularity, and bone mineral density in female runners. Med Sci Sports Exerc 2003;35(5):711–9.

[60] Beck TJ, Ruff CB, Mourtada FA, et al. Dual-energy X-ray absorptiometry derived structural geometry for stress fracture prediction in male US Marine Corps recruits. J Bone Miner Res 1996;11(5):645–53.

[61] Milgrom C, Giladi M, Simkin A, et al. An analysis of the biomechanical mechanism of tibial stress fractures among Israeli infantry recruits. A prospective study. Clin Orthop 1988;(231):216–21.

[62] Milgrom C, Giladi M, Simkin A, et al. The area moment of inertia of the tibia: a risk factor for stress fractures. J Biomech 1989;22(11–12):1243–8.

[63] Giladi M, Milgrom C, Simkin A, et al. Stress fractures and tibial bone width. A risk factor. J Bone Joint Surg Br 1987;69(2):326–9.

[64] Miller GJ, Purkey WW Jr. The geometric properties of paired human tibiae. J Biomech 1980;13(1):1–8.

[65] Giladi M, Milgrom C, Stein M. The low arch, a protective factor in stress fractures. A prospective study of 295 military recruits. Orthop Rev 1985;(14):709–12.

[66] Simkin A, Leichter I, Giladi M, et al. Combined effect of foot arch structure and an orthotic device on stress fractures. Foot Ankle 1989;10(1):25–9.

[67] Friberg O. Leg length asymmetry in stress fractures. A clinical and radiological study. J Sports Med Phys Fitness 1982;22(4):485–8.

[68] Cowan DN, Jones BH, Frykman PN, et al. Lower limb morphology and risk of overuse injury among male infantry trainees. Med Sci Sports Exerc 1996;28(8):945–52.

[69] Finestone A, Shlamkovitch N, Eldad A, et al. Risk factors for stress fractures among Israeli infantry recruits. Mil Med 1991;156(10):528–30.

[70] Stager JM, Hatler LK. Menarche in athletes: the influence of genetics and prepubertal training. Med Sci Sports Exerc 1988;20(4):369–73.

[71] Warren MP, Brooks-Gunn J, Hamilton LH, et al. Scoliosis and fractures in young ballet dancers. Relation to delayed menarche and secondary amenorrhea. N Engl J Med 1986; 314(21):1348–53.

[72] Loucks AB, Horvath SM. Athletic amenorrhea: a review. Med Sci Sports Exerc 1985;17(1): 56–72.

[73] Drinkwater BL, Nilson K, Chesnut CH, et al. Bone mineral content of amenorrheic and eumenorrheic athletes. N Engl J Med 1984;311(5):277–81.

[74] Frost HM. A new direction for osteoporosis research: a review and proposal. Bone 1991; 12(6):429–37.

[75] Bennell KL, Malcolm SA, Thomas SA, et al. Risk factors for stress fractures in female track-and-field athletes: a retrospective analysis. Clin J Sport Med 1995;5(4):229–35.

[76] Hergenroeder AC. Bone mineralization, hypothalamic amenorrhea, and sex steroid therapy in female adolescents and young adults. J Pediatr 1995;126(5)(Pt 1):683–9.

[77] Cumming DC, Wall SR, Galbraith MA, et al. Reproductive hormone responses to resistance exercise. Med Sci Sports Exerc 1987;19(3):234–8.

[78] Klibanski A, Biller BM, Schoenfeld DA, et al. The effects of estrogen administration on trabecular bone loss in young women with anorexia nervosa. J Clin Endocrinol Metab 1995;80(3):898–904.

[79] Warren MP, Perlroth NE. The effects of intense exercise on the female reproductive system. J Endocrinol 2001;170(1):3–11.

[80] Seeman E, Szmukler GI, Formica C, et al. Osteoporosis in anorexia nervosa: the influence of peak bone density, bone loss, oral contraceptive use, and exercise. J Bone Miner Res 1992;7(12):1467–74.

[81] Hartard M, Kleinmond C, Kirchbichler A, et al. Age at first oral contraceptive use as a major determinant of vertebral bone mass in female endurance athletes. Bone 2004;35(4): 836–41.

[82] Berenson AB, Radecki CM, Grady JJ, et al. A prospective, controlled study of the effects of hormonal contraception on bone mineral density. Obstet Gynecol 2001;98(4):576–82.

[83] Specker BL. Evidence for an interaction between calcium intake and physical activity on changes in bone mineral density. J Bone Miner Res 1996;11(10):1539–44.

[84] Bennell K, Matheson G, Meeuwisse W, et al. Risk factors for stress fractures. Sports Med 1999;28(2):91–122.

[85] Cooper KL, Beabout JW, Swee RG. Insufficiency fractures of the sacrum. Radiology 1985; 156(1):15–20.

[86] Eisman JA. Vitamin D receptor gene alleles and osteoporosis: an affirmative view. J Bone Miner Res 1995;10(9):1289–93.

[87] Fleet JC, Harris SS, Wood RJ, et al. The BsmI vitamin D receptor restriction fragment length polymorphism (BB) predicts low bone density in premenopausal black and white women. J Bone Miner Res 1995;10(6):985–90.

[88] Morrison NA, Qi JC, Tokita A, et al. Prediction of bone density from vitamin D receptor alleles. Nature 1994;367(6460):284–7.

[89] Rigotti NA, Nussbaum SR, Herzog DB, et al. Osteoporosis in women with anorexia nervosa. N Engl J Med 1984;311(25):1601–6.

[90] Bachrach LK, Guido D, Katzman D, et al. Decreased bone density in adolescent girls with anorexia nervosa. Pediatrics 1990;86(3):440–7.

[91] Frusztajer NT, Dhuper S, Warren MP, et al. Nutrition and the incidence of stress fractures in ballet dancers. Am J Clin Nutr 1990;51(5):779–83.

[92] Nattiv A, Puffer JC, Green GA. Lifestyles and health risks of collegiate athletes: a multi-center study. Clin J Sport Med 1997;7(4):262–72.

[93] Hoch AZ, Dempsey RL, Carrera GF, et al. Is there an association between athletic amenorrhea and endothelial cell dysfunction? Med Sci Sports Exerc 2003;35(3):377–83.

[94] Nattiv A, Agostini R, Drinkwater B, et al. The female athlete triad. The inter-relatedness of disordered eating, amenorrhea, and osteoporosis. Clin Sports Med 1994;13(2):405–18.

[95] Loucks AB. Energy availability, not body fatness, regulates reproductive function in women. Exerc Sport Sci Rev 2003;31(3):144–8.

[96] Slemenda CW, Reister TK, Hui SL, et al. Influences on skeletal mineralization in children and adolescents: evidence for varying effects of sexual maturation and physical activity. J Pediatr 1994;125(2):201–7.

[97] Writing Group for the ISCD Position Development Conference. Diagnosis of osteoporosis in men, premenopausal women, and children. J Clin Densitom 2004;7(1):17–26.

[98] Sullivan D, Warren RF, Pavlov H, et al. Stress fractures in 51 runners. Clin Orthop 1984;(187):188–92.

[99] Miller C, Major N, Toth A. Pelvic stress injuries in the athlete: management and prevention. Sports Med 2003;33(13):1003–12.

[100] Ishibashi Y, Okamura Y, Otsuka H, et al. Comparison of scintigraphy and magnetic resonance imaging for stress injuries of bone. Clin J Sport Med 2002;12(2):79–84.

[101] Brukner P. Exercise-related lower leg pain: bone. Med Sci Sports Exerc 2000;32(3 Suppl): S15–26.

[102] Boam WD, Miser WF, Yuill SC, et al. Comparison of ultrasound examination with bone scintiscan in the diagnosis of stress fractures. J Am Board Fam Pract 1996;9(6):414–7.

[103] Swenson EJ Jr, DeHaven KE, Sebastianelli WJ, et al. The effect of a pneumatic leg brace on return to play in athletes with tibial stress fractures. Am J Sports Med 1997;25(3):322–8.

[104] Benazzo F, Mosconi M, Beccarisi G, et al. Use of capacitive coupled electric fields in stress fractures in athletes. Clin Orthop 1995;(310):145–9.

[105] Verma RB, Sherman O. Athletic stress fractures: part I. History, epidemiology, physiology, risk factors, radiography, diagnosis, and treatment. Am J Orthop 2001;30(11):798–806.

[106] Fredericson M, Bergman AG, Matheson GO. [Stress fractures in athletes]. Orthopade 1997;26:961–71 [in German].

[107] Arendt E, Griffin LY. Musculoskeletal injuries. In: Drinkwater BL, editor. Women in sport. Oxford (UK): Blackwell Science; 2000. p. 208–40.

[108] Almeida SA, Trone DW, Leone DM, et al. Gender differences in musculoskeletal injury rates: a function of symptom reporting? Med Sci Sports Exerc 1999;31(12):1807–12.

[109] Heintjes E, Berger MY, Bierma-Zeinstra SM, et al. Exercise therapy for patellofemoral pain syndrome. Cochrane Database Syst Rev 2003;4:CD003472.

[110] Dye SF, Vaupel GL, Dye CC. Conscious neurosensory mapping of the internal structures of the human knee without intraarticular anesthesia. Am J Sports Med 1998;26(6):773–7.

[111] Duri ZA, Patel DV, Aichroth PM. The immature athlete. Clin Sports Med 2002;21(3): 461–82.

[112] Fredericson M. Common injuries in runners. Diagnosis, rehabilitation and prevention. Sports Med 1996;21(1):49–72.

[113] Heintjes E, Berger MY, Bierma-Zeinstra SM, et al. Pharmacotherapy for patellofemoral pain syndrome. Cochrane Database Syst Rev 2004;CD003470.

[114] Crossley K, Bennell K, Green S, et al. Physical therapy for patellofemoral pain. Am J Sports Med 2002;30(6):857–65.

[115] Cowan SM, Bennell KL, Hodges PW, et al. Delayed onset of electromyographic activity of vastus medialis obliquus relative to vastus lateralis in subjects with patellofemoral pain syndrome. Arch Phys Med Rehabil 2001;82(2):183–9.

[116] Cerny K. Vastus medialis oblique/vastus lateralis muscle activity ratios for selected exercises in persons with and without patellofemoral pain syndrome. Phys Ther 1995;75(8): 672–83.

[117] Powers CM. Rehabilitation of patellofemoral joint disorders: a critical review. J Orthop Sports Phys Ther 1998;28(5):345–54.

[118] Cowan SM, Bennell K, Hodges PW. Therapeutic patellar taping changes the timing of vasti muscle activation in people with patellofemoral pain syndrome. Clin J Sport Med 2002;12: 339–47.
[119] Cowan SM, Bennell KL, Crossley KM, et al. Physical therapy for patellofemoral pain: a randomized, double-blinded, placebo-controlled trial. Med Sci Sports Exerc 2002;34(12): 1879–85.
[120] Fredericson M, Powers CM. Practical management of patellofemoral pain. Clin J Sport Med 2002;12(1):36–8.
[121] D'Hondt NE, Struijs PA, Kerkhoffs GM, et al. Orthotic devices for treating patellofemoral pain syndrome. Cochrane Database Syst Rev 2002(2):CD002267.
[122] Hertel J, Sloss BR, Earl JE. Effect of foot orthotics on quadriceps and gluteus medius electromyographic activity during selected exercises. Arch Phys Med Rehabil 2005;86(1): 26–30.
[123] Gross MT, Foxworth JL. The role of foot orthoses as an intervention for patellofemoral pain. J Orthop Sports Phys Ther 2003;33(11):661–70.
[124] Fulkerson JP. Diagnosis and treatment of patients with patellofemoral pain. Am J Sports Med 2002;30(3):447–56.
[125] Fredericson M, White JJ, Macmahon JM, et al. Quantitative analysis of the relative effectiveness of 3 iliotibial band stretches. Arch Phys Med Rehabil 2002;83(5):589–92.
[126] Akuthota V, Stilp S, Lento P. Iliotibial band syndrome. In: Frontera W, Silver J, editors. Essentials of physical medicine and rehabilitation. Philadelphia: Hanley and Belfus; 2002. p. 328–33.
[127] Fredericson M, Cookingham CL, Chaudhari AM, et al. Hip abductor weakness in distance runners with iliotibial band syndrome. Clin J Sport Med 2000;10(3):169–75.

ELSEVIER
SAUNDERS

Phys Med Rehabil Clin N Am
16 (2005) 779–799

PHYSICAL MEDICINE
AND REHABILITATION
CLINICS OF
NORTH AMERICA

# Evidence-Based Treatment of Foot and Ankle Injuries in Runners

## Karen P. Barr, MD[a],*, Mark A. Harrast, MD[a,b]

[a]Department of Rehabilitation Medicine, Box 356490, University of Washington,
Seattle, WA 98195, USA
[b]Department of Orthopaedics and Sports Medicine, Box 356490, University of Washington,
Seattle, WA 98195, USA

## Foot injuries

### Epidemiology

Forty to 50% of all running injuries occur below the knee. Between 10% and 20% of all running injuries are foot injuries. Foot problems are the most common injuries that are reported by long distance and marathon runners [1,2]. There are several reasons why foot injuries are so common. One is the high prevalence of foot pain in the general population, not just runners. The incidence of foot problems is as high as 80% in the general population [3]. The other reason is the great biomechanical stress that is placed on the foot during running.

The foot is the only structure of the body that regularly contacts the ground. It consists of bones, tendons, and ligaments, without prominent muscle mass, so it is different from other areas that usually are addressed in sports medicine, and different rehabilitation principles apply. This bony and ligamentous structure must withstand ground reaction forces during running that are equal to three to four times normal body weight [4]. In addition to the increase in the amount of force during running, there is increased demand for this to occur efficiently and with optimal neuromuscular coordination. During running, the stance phase of gait changes from about 60% of the gait cycle to as little as 30%. During this shortened stance phase there is increased demands on the foot because it must change rapidly from a rigid structure at initial contact with the ground to prevent buckling of the knee, to the planted foot which needs to be flexible to accommodate uneven surfaces and allow the forces to be dispersed over a broader surface

---

* Corresponding author.
*E-mail address:* barrk@u.washington.edu (K.P. Barr).

area, and then back to a rigid structure to transfer forces during push off [5]. The unique structure of the foot allows it to accommodate to these increasing demands; however, common training errors, such as rapid increase in mileage or training intensity, poor footwear, and functional or structural faults, can lead to injury of a variety of structures.

## Anatomy and biomechanics of the foot

The foot has a complex structure. For clinical discussions, it usually is divided into three distinct regions: (1) the rearfoot, which consists of the calcaneus and talus and related soft tissue structures; (2) the midfoot, which consists of the cuneiforms, the navicular, and the cuboid and related soft tissue structures; and (3) the forefoot, which consists of the metatarsals and phalanges [6].

The rearfoot is involved with the tibiofibular joint and the talocrural joint (see later discussion) and the subtalar joint, between the calcaneus and talus, which is a key structure that is critical to function of the rearfoot. The subtalar joint has three degrees of freedom and allows motion in several planes at once. This allows the foot to adapt to sloping and uneven terrain and to transmit forces efficiently. At heel strike, the subtalar joint is in supination which allows the hind and midfoot to be in a locked position, and therefore, act more like a rigid lever. The subtalar joint moves into pronation to assist the ankle and knee with impact shock absorption and to adapt better to ground surfaces. This allows the foot to be a mobile, adaptive structure. Then, as the body crosses over the foot, the joint moves back into supination to increase the rigidity of the structure for push off. Excessive or delayed motion at this joint is believed to be a major factor in running injuries of the lower limb [4,5,7].

The midfoot makes the "keystones" of the foot arches. The medially-located navicular bone provides stability for the medial longitudinal arch. The laterally-located cuboid provides stability for the lateral longitudinal arch, and the cuneiforms in the middle make up the transverse arch. In isolation, these midfoot joints allow only minimal movement; however, taken together, they allow for significant movement to enable the foot to adapt to many different positions. Together, the joints in this area are known as Chopart's joints. These joints also move from a rigid phase to an unlocked phase during the gait cycle. Common running injuries in this area are due to stress fractures and injuries to the many ligaments that attach in this region of the foot.

The forefoot begins at the tarsometatarsal joints, which also are known as Lisfranc's joints [3]. The first, second, and third metatarsals articulate with their associated cuneiform. The shape of the most medial cuneiform determines the mobility of the first ray, which many investigators believe is an important contributor to running injuries of the foot. The base of the second metatarsal is in a recessed position as it articulates with the second cuneiform; this makes it inherently more rigid than its neighbors, and thus, is more susceptible to stress fractures in runners. The fourth metatarsal also is stable. The fifth metatarsal is more mobile [7], and so is a less common site of stress fractures; however; when fractures do occur, healing may be delayed and close attention is necessary because of the increased mobility in this area [6]. At the end of the stance phase, the metatarsal phalangeal joints are extended fully. This creates tautness of the plantar fascia and elevation and rigidity of the longitudinal arch. This is called the windlass mechanism and stabilizes the foot during push off [5].

## Foot injuries

Common foot injuries in runners include tendinopathies, stress fractures, and a variety of soft tissue injuries. Injuries to be aware of are nerve entrapments and other neurologic injuries, and manifestations of systemic diseases. A regional approach to the differential diagnosis of running injuries of the foot is outlined below. Evidence-based medicine is discussed when it is available, and the rehabilitation approach to treatment is detailed.

## Rearfoot pain

### Plantar fasciitis

Plantar fasciitis is the most common cause of rearfoot pain in runners. The diagnosis usually is made clinically. Patients present with gradual onset of pain in the inferior heel, which is worse in the first few steps in the morning or after rest. It also may worsen by the end of the day or after a run because of fatigue. Like other overuse injuries, symptoms usually are preceded by training errors [8]. On physical examination, there is point tenderness over the anteromedial aspect of the heel at the medial process of the calcaneal tuberosity. A less painful, but still tender, area is along the plantar fascia, particularly the medial part. Symptoms usually worsen with passive dorsiflexion of the toes. Limited foot dorsiflexion usually is seen. A study of 50 consecutive patients who were referred to physical therapy for plantar fasciitis compared risk factors of the patients with a group of age-matched controls; limited dorsiflexion on the involved side significantly increased the risk for plantar fasciitis. This relationship was exponential. Ankle dorsiflexion of 6° to 10° had an odds ratio of 2.9, whereas those who had 0° or less of dorsiflexion had an odds ratio of 23.3. Increased body mass index also increased the risk for plantar fasciitis [9]. In a large study of runners who had injuries, older age and heavier weight were associated with plantar fasciitis [2]. Regarding foot structure, excessive pronation and supination have been blamed as causes of plantar fasciitis [7].

The rest of the physical examination rules out competing diagnoses for heel pain. Enthesopathies and heel pain is a common complaint in patients who have spondyloarthropathies, so this should not be missed. Other common diagnoses that are seen in runners are discussed below.

Imaging is not needed, except to rule out other diagnoses. Often, a heel spur is seen on radiograph which most likely is a result of increased forces that are caused by the tight fascia and abnormal biomechanics, and is not a cause of the pain [6].

Treatment usually is successful with a combination of symptom control and improving biomechanics. Pain almost always is controlled by decreasing running, ice to the fascia, nonsteroidal anti-inflammatory drugs (NSAIDs), and cross-friction massage. The main biomechanical problem is decreased dorsiflexion, so stretching of the gastroc-soleus complex is key. Stretching of the plantar fascia by dorsiflexing the toes and the foot at the same time also is indicated. A prospective randomized study of 100 patients who had chronic plantar fasciitis of at least 10 months duration compared a group performing standard weight-bearing Achilles stretching with a group that stretched the plantar fascia by manually applying overpressure to their dorsiflexed toes and ankles while sitting. Both groups received an over-the-counter soft shoe insert and took NSAIDs for 3 weeks. Both groups had an improvement in pain and function, but the group that did the plantar fascia stretching improved more [10]. The second most common biomechanical problem is weakness of the plantar flexors. Failure in eccentric loading allows increased forces to be transmitted to the insertion of the fascia. Therefore, strengthening, especially eccentric strengthening, is important. The other common deficits that are seen include poor balance and gluteus medius weakness, which can be addressed with a proper exercise program [11].

If symptoms do not improve with physical therapy and medication, orthotics and heel pads often are prescribed. In a study of 236 patients, all of whom received stretching exercises, four different shoe inserts were compared: a silicone heel pad, a rubber insert, a felt pad, and a custom orthosis. Those with the silicone insert improved the most, whereas those with the custom orthoses improved the least. The group that had the custom orthoses did worse than the group that did stretching alone [12]. Other studies that used heel pads and soft-molded orthoses found them to be helpful as well [13]. Magnetic insoles did not have any benefit over regular cushioned insoles [14].

For resistant cases, some have advocated night splints that dorsiflex the ankle at bedtime and provide a prolonged stretch. Several small, randomized controlled trials showed superior outcomes with this treatment in patients who complied with wearing the splints [15], but other studies did not find them to be effective [8].

Shock wave therapy for chronic plantar fasciitis also has been the subject of several recent randomized controlled trials. This is indicated only if the patient has failed the above outlined treatments. There is no consensus at this time as to whether repeated low-energy shock wave therapy, which does not require anesthesia, or single high-energy shock waves, which requires local or regional anesthesia (usually an ankle block), is superior. In a study of runners who had plantar fasciitis who ran at least 30 miles per week before injury and in whom conservative treatment had failed, low-energy extracorporeal shock wave therapy was compared with sham therapy. They found a significant reduction of pain first thing in the morning; pain ratings decreased from an average of 7 to 2 in the treatment group and 7 to 5 in the sham group at 6 months. Sixty percent of the treatment group versus 27% of the sham group had greater than 50% improvement at 6 months [16]. Similarly positive results have been found with high-energy shock wave treatments [17].

Corticosteroid injection into the most tender area of the plantar fascia also is a common treatment for this condition. A study that evaluated this treatment was limited by low follow-up responses, but revealed significant pain relief at 1 month, but no difference at 3 to 6 months. Clinicians worry that steroid injections weaken the fascia and could result in increased risk for rupture, but this has not been proven in the literature [8].

## Fat pad contusions and pain

Fat pad contusions and atrophy are another common cause of heel pain. It has not been as well studied as plantar fasciitis. A heel cushion is the usual treatment.

## Calcaneal and talar stress fractures

These are not nearly as common as mid- and forefoot stress fractures (see later discussion). Little research has been done in this area. Patients present with heel pain with running or walking that is relieved with nonweightbearing. Imaging with bone scan, CT, or MRI confirms the diagnosis. Treatment is the same as outlined below for other stress fractures.

## Tarsal tunnel syndrome

This is entrapment of the tibial nerve as it passes behind the medial malleolus. It is much more likely to occur after trauma to the ankle than spontaneously or with overuse, but these can be mechanisms of injury as well, especially in runners who pronate excessively. Any or all of the branches of the tibial nerve in the foot may be involved. Patients present with deep aching pain and paresthesias in the plantar surface of the foot. Symptoms may worsen with running or at night. On physical examination, a Tinel's sign at the area of entrapment may be positive. Pain may be provoked by forceful active pronation or by sustained passive eversion, because both of these stress the area [6,18]. It is rare to find true neurologic loss, such as intrinsic foot muscle wasting or weakness or dense sensory loss. Neurologic examination should rule out competing diagnoses, such as peripheral neuropathy or radiculopathy. Electrodiagnostic studies will confirm the diagnosis. Treatment includes correcting biomechanical problems and ankle rehabilitation, such as Achilles stretching and proprioceptive training. If this is not successful, steroid injections and surgery are other modes of treatment [19].

## Midfoot pain

### Navicular stress fractures

This is a common stress fracture in runners, so it should be ruled out in any runner who presents with vague midfoot pain. The differential diagnosis includes extensor tendinopathy, which usually is more tender to palpation on the plantar surface and with resisted foot dorsiflexion, and midtarsal joint sprains, which usually are associated with a discrete event, such as twisting the foot or tripping. With a navicular stress fracture, physical examination is remarkable for tenderness directly over the bone when the proximal dorsal surface is palpated (often called the "N spot"). Pain is made worse by hopping. It is diagnosed definitively by bone scan, MRI, or CT. There can be a long recovery with prolonged time off from running. Treatment begins with 6 weeks of nonweightbearing, with gradual return to sport.

### Posterior tibial tendinopathy

The posterior tibial tendon passes behind the medial malleolus and inserts on the navicular bone. Injury of this tendon can cause ankle and midfoot pain. It is a common overuse injury that is seen with rapid increases in training intensity or poor footwear because of the eccentric forces that occur as the posterior tibial muscle resists descent of the medial longitudinal arch. Runners present with tenderness along the tendon from the ankle to the midfoot and pain with resisted foot inversion. On physical examination, excessive pronation and a tight posterior tibialis muscle usually are found. Rehabilitation consists of addressing these issues, potentially with an orthosis, as well as the usual care of tendon disorders.

### Peroneal tendinopathy

The peroneal tendons pass behind the lateral malleolus, where they can be a source of pain, and then diverge so that the peroneus brevis tendon can insert on the base of the fifth metatarsal; the peroneus longus runs deep across the foot through a groove in the cuboid to insert onto the base of the first metatarsal and medial cuneiform [20]. The tendon can be a source of pain anywhere along this course, and symptoms are aggravated by resisted eversion and plantarflexion. It is associated with excessive pronation at toe off, and weak plantarflexion, so these should be addressed in the treatment phase [7].

### Anterior tarsal tunnel syndrome

This is entrapment of the deep peroneal nerve as it passes under the extensor retinaculum. Patients present with aching and numbness on the dorsum of the midfoot, which can extend to the first web space. It is believed to be caused most commonly by poor fitting shoes, so may respond to changes in footwear. Other treatments that are used often include corticosteroid injections, ankle rehabilitation, and surgical release.

## Forefoot pain

### Metatarsal stress fractures

Stress fractures are common overuse injuries in runners, with a prevalence as high as 9% in collegiate runners. They are more common in women. A retrospective study that examined 10 years of injuries to collegiate athletes in several sports found that distance runners were most likely to sustain a stress fracture. Foot stress fractures were the most common type that were seen in runners in this study; they were divided equally between navicular and metatarsal fractures [21]. Other studies of running injuries found high percentages of stress fractures of the foot [22,23], especially metatarsal fractures that involved the second and third metatarsals. The second metatarsal is particularly vulnerable because the proximal head is tucked between the medial and lateral cuneiforms and is immobile [5]. Fifth metatarsal stress fractures are uncommon in runners, but may be more difficult to treat. If the fracture occurs at the diaphysis, it is known as a Jones fracture, and requires prolonged nonweightbearing; it may require surgery if nonunion occurs [6].

Biomechanical risk factors for foot fractures have been examined. In a Finnish study of elite runners who had recurrent stress fractures, a relationship between a high longitudinal arch and cavus-type foot and stress fractures was found. Similar results were found in other studies, particularly studies of military recruits who suffered stress fractures of the foot. This is believed to be secondary to the more rigid, reduced shock absorbency of this type of foot [5,24]. Other investigators believe that a pes planus foot is more at risk because of increased pronation, and therefore, muscular fatigue, which causes increased forces to be transmitted to the bone [1,7,24]. Other commonly cited risk factors are high mileage, sudden escalation of mileage, training on hard surfaces, and nonmenstruation in women [1,21,24].

Patients usually present with foot pain that is worse with running and better with rest. At first, symptoms may be intermittent, but begin to occur with all activity. They often present 4 to 5 weeks after a sudden training increase. The most common physical examination finding is point tenderness over the fracture. Imaging confirms the diagnosis. Plain films can remain normal for 3 to 6 weeks after symptoms develop. The first change seen is subperiosteal bone formation. Sometimes changes are never seen on plain films [7]. Bone scans will be positive in 20% to 40% of cases in which clinical suspicion is high but plain films are normal [21]. MRI also is sensitive in showing stress fractures. Some investigators believe that MRI is too sensitive, because it sometimes shows bony reaction in asymptomatic athletes. Grading scales have been developed for MRI changes that correlate with prognosis [21].

There are no good randomized controlled trials that evaluated treatment for stress fractures of the metatarsals. Generally, treatment begins with reducing activity to a pain-free level; therefore, if walking is painful, the patient should be made nonweightbearing, but if walking is not painful, it is permitted. Rehabilitation begins with swimming or pool running so that aerobic fitness can be maintained. Muscle imbalances and inflexibilities of the lower extremities are addressed, depending on the individual needs of the patient. After they can do the activity pain-free, patients may progress to nonpounding upright activity, such as cycling, elliptical training, or Stairmaster machines, and lower extremity weight training. Gradually, running and sports drills are added and then time and distance is increased gradually as long as the patient remains asymptomatic. Orthotics may be prescribed to accommodate a less than ideal foot structure. In female athletes, general bone health and hormonal issues may need to be explored.

Return to full running is variable, depending on the grade of the fracture and the patient's healing capacity. In a study of collegiate athletes in a wide variety of sports who had various stress fractures, the average return to sport was 8.4 weeks [21].

*Metatarsalgia*

This is a common condition in runners to consider after metatarsal stress fractures are ruled out. Patients complain of pain on the plantar surface of the metatarsal heads that is worse with running and better at rest. Tenderness in this area is found on physical examination. Often, an overpronated foot is seen. This is because the first and second metatarsal heads may accept increased force at impact because of the excessive pronation [5]. It is treated by a metatarsal pad that is placed proximal to the painful area to relieve pressure on the metatarsals and spread forces over a larger area, or a custom orthosis that can provide the same function along with a cut-out for the painful metatarsal head to relieve pressure further.

*Extensor and flexor tendonitis*

Forefoot tendonitis, especially extensor tendonitis, is common in runners. Running hills is believed to be a risk factor because of the challenge to toe dorsiflexion range of motion (ROM) when running uphill, and the challenge of a prolonged eccentric contraction when running downhill [7]. Treatment is the same as for other tendon injuries—relieve pressure to the area by not overtightening shoe laces, decrease pain with NSAIDs and ice, and address strength and flexibility deficits of the foot and ankle.

*First metatarsal phalangeal conditions*

Running can aggravate common conditions of the first metatarsal phalangeal, such as hallux rigidis and hallux valgus. Generally, these are managed with activity modification and orthoses in runners who want to pursue conservative care and continue to run. Hallucis sesamoids also can be aggravated by running, especially sprinting. Patients have pain with weight bearing and walking. Physical examination reveals tenderness and swelling in the area. Often, it is difficult to differentiate stress fractures of the sesamoid from sesamoiditis, which is pain and swelling of the tendon around the sesamoids. These injuries are difficult to treat and may require prolonged rest and unweighting the area with orthoses or padding [6].

*Interdigital neuromas*

Symptoms are caused by swelling of the nerves and scar tissue around the nerves. This is believed to be secondary to repetitive toe dorsiflexion that occurs at push off during running and excessive foot pronation. Patients complain of numbness and pain in the toes that is worse with tight shoes and when weight is placed through the forefoot. The third intermetatarsal space is affected most commonly, so the third and fourth toes are numb most commonly [18]. Treatment is usually with metatarsal pads, widened footwear, and strengthening of foot intrinsics. In some cases, surgery is necessary to relieve symptoms.

## Ankle injuries

*Epidemiology*

The ankle is another area that is injured commonly in running, and in sports that require running. Ankle injuries account for approximately 15% of all sports injuries [25]. Like foot injuries, ankle injuries can be divided into overuse injuries and traumatic injuries. Overuse injuries in the ankle usually are tendon injuries, the most common of which is Achilles tendinopathy. By far, the most common traumatic injury is a lateral ankle sprain. Other, less common injuries of the ankle also are discussed below.

*Anatomy and biomechanics of the ankle*

The ankle consists of the talocrural joint and the distal tibiofibular joint. The talocrural articulation is a hinged synovial joint that is located between the distal tibia and fibula and the superior portion of the talus. The distal tibiofibular articulation is a fibrous joint, or syndesmosis. A strong interosseous ligament forms the principle connection between the tibia and fibula at this joint. The anterior and posterior tibiofibular ligaments provide further supports to this joint.

The superior surface of the talus, or trochlea, is pulley-shaped and bears the weight of the body that is transmitted by way of the tibia. The body of the talus has three continuous facets for articulations superiorly with the tibia, laterally with the medial malleolus, and medially with the lateral malleolus. The inferior surface of the talus articulates with the calcaneus. Posteriorly, the talus has medial and lateral tubercles that form a grove in between for the flexor hallucis longus tendon to pass into the foot. During ossification, the lateral tubercle may fail to unite with the body of the talus;

this results in an extra bone, the os trigonum. Finally, the talus articulates anteriorly with the navicular.

Dorsiflexion and plantarflexion are the primary movements of the talocrural joint. During plantarflexion, some rotation and abduction/ adduction can occur. In dorsiflexion and the neutral position, the ankle is stable given its bony articulations which are supported by powerful ligaments and are crossed by several tendons which are bound tightly down by a retinacula, or thickened deep fascia. During plantarflexion, however, the trochlea of the talus moves anteriorly in the tibial mortise; this lessens bony stability and creates more reliance on the ligamentous contribution.

The fibrous capsule of the talocrural joint is reinforced medially by the deltoid ligament and laterally by the lateral ligaments. The deltoid ligament attaches the medial malleolus to the talus, navicular, and calcaneus. It also helps to support the medial longitudinal arch. This ligamentous complex consists of four parts: tibionavicular, anterior and posterior tibiotalar, and tibiocalcaneal ligaments. The ligaments rarely are injured because the complex is strong and eversion injuries are less common.

The three lateral ligaments, which are not as strong as the deltoid ligament, attach the lateral malleolus to the talus and calcaneus. They are named the anterior talofibular ligament (ATFL), the calcaneofibular ligament (CFL), and posterior talofibular ligament (PTFL). The ATFL primarily prevents anterior translation of the talus on the tibial mortise; however, in plantarflexion, the ligament's orientation allows it to prevent inversion. It is the weakest of the lateral ligaments, and thus, is the one that is injured most commonly. The CFL prevents inversion at the talocrural and the subtalar (talocalcaneal) joints. The PTFL prevents posterior talar translation on the tibia. It is the strongest of the lateral ligaments and is taut only in extreme dorsiflexion; therefore, it is only injured in severe ankle sprains.

Regarding the muscles that act on the ankle, the main dorsiflexors are the tibialis anterior and extensor digitorum longus, although the extensor hallucis longus and peroneus tertius can assist. The chief plantarflexors include the gastrocnemius and soleus, but are assisted by the plantaris, tibialis posterior, flexor hallucis longus, and flexor digitorum longus.

*Ankle injuries*

Common ankle injuries in runners primarily include tendinopathies and ligamentous sprains; however, osteochondral injuries, nerve entrapments, and other neurologic injuries must remain on the differential diagnosis when evaluating a runner who has an ankle injury. Differentiating the far more common overuse, insidious injuries from acute, traumatic injuries also is important. A regional approach to the differential diagnosis of ankle injuries in runners is outlined below. Evidence-based treatment with a focus on rehabilitation is highlighted. Lateral ankle ligamentous sprains and Achilles tendinopathy are paid specific attention as prototypes of treatment protocols for ankle injuries in runners.

## Lateral ankle pain

### Ligamentous sprains

Although more insidious/overuse injuries are more common in runners, they also can sustain acute trauma. Lateral ankle sprains are one of the most common sports-related injuries; cross-country running probably is the most risky for the runner [26]. More than 40% of ankle sprains can progress to chronic problems [27]. In runners, ankle sprains occur more commonly in adolescents. Inversion injuries are most common, thus straining the lateral ligaments. These are more common because the lateral malleolus projects more distally (than the medial) which creates a bony block to significant eversion.

Because the typical mechanism of injury is inversion, supination, and plantarflexion of the foot while the tibia rotates externally, there is a predictable sequence of ligamentous tears [27]. The ATFL is damaged before the CFL. The PTFL is damaged only in severe injuries and frequently is associated with a fracture. The ATFL is an intracapsular structure, and thus, if torn, hemarthrosis can result. Ligament injuries are graded in severity from I to III. A grade I injury involves ligamentous stretching but no gross tears. A grade II injury involves partial ligamentous tearing, whereas a grade III injury involves a complete ligamentous rupture. It is important to grade these injuries correctly because it aids in prognosis and determining the appropriate rehabilitation. Eighty-six percent of ankle ligament tears are midsubstance, and thus, only 14% are avulsion injuries [27]. Sixty-five percent of grade III sprains are solely ATFL tears and 20% include the ATFL and the CFL [27].

When taking a history of a runner who has ankle pain, it is important to understand the mechanism of injury, which can clue the practitioner to the injured structures. The locations of pain and swelling also help to determine the site of injury. Determining the onset of pain is helpful in that a runner who can bear weight immediately following the injury and then develops pain and swelling as he continues to run suggests a ligamentous injury over a fracture and also can help to indicate the severity of injury; continuing to run is an indication that little to no instability is present.

The examination of the runner who has a suspected ankle sprain begins with observation that specifically looks for swelling, ecchymosis, and any deformity while standing (if possible) and supine. Palpating for the exact location of tenderness can help to establish if the injury is solely ligamentous or if a fracture may be involved. Be certain to palpate the ligaments, malleoli, talus, distal and proximal fibula, base of the fifth metatarsal, and the peroneal tendon. Assess active and passive ankle ROM. Plantarflexion typically exacerbates pain by stressing the ATFL. Assess the runner's neurovascular status by palpating the pedal arteries and testing sensation in the sural and peroneal nerves' distribution.

Provocative maneuvers include the anterior drawer and talar tilt tests. The anterior drawer estimates ATFL stability [28]. The examiner attempts to translate the foot anterior to the tibia while gripping the heal. The runner's knee should be flexed to relax the gastrocnemius. Test reliability, however, is poor, partially because of patient guarding secondary to pain.

The talar tilt, or inversion, test estimates CFL integrity [29]. The ankle is grasped and moved into inversion to assess the motion of the talus and calcaneus on the tibia and fibula. This test is difficult when examining an acute injury because of pain and swelling. van Dijk et al [30] recommended that the physical examination be delayed for 4 to 5 days after the initial injury to improve its sensitivity and specificity.

Radiography in evaluating ankle sprains is guided by the Ottawa Ankle Rules [31]. These state that ankle films should be taken if there is bony tenderness in the posterior half of the lower 6 cm of the tibia or fibula or an inability to bear weight immediately after injury and during the clinical assessment. Foot radiographs are indicated if the athlete has bony tenderness over the fifth metatarsal or navicular or if there is an inability to bear weight immediately after injury and during the clinical assessment. If the athlete presents within 10 days of injury, no significant fracture has been missed with these guidelines. Standard ankle films include anteroposterior (AP), lateral, and mortise views. The mortise projection is an AP view with the leg internally rotated 20° to allow the beam to be perpendicular to the intermalleolar line. Stress radiography is not used commonly because it does not detect an injury reliably [32]. MRI is used rarely in the setting of acute ankle sprains; however, it can be helpful in the evaluation of chronic ankle sprains or ankle pain that is not relieved with regular conservative measures to evaluate for talar dome lesions, other osteochondral injuries, or peroneal tendon involvement. Injuries to the talar dome occur in 7% to 22% of ankle sprains and are missed commonly on initial evaluation [33].

Initial management of an ankle sprain involves controlling pain and swelling and maintaining ROM. PRICE (protection, rest, ice, compression, and elevation) is appropriate to start. Cryotherapy helps to reduce effusion and potentially decreases metabolism which may limit secondary hypoxic injury [34]. Hocutt [35] et al demonstrated better outcomes in patients who started cryotherapy within 36 hours of injury. Wrapping the acutely injured ankle with an elastic bandage, distal to proximal, also can minimize effusion. Use of electrical stimulation and ultrasound have not demonstrated a definite reduction in swelling with human subjects, although they may be helpful for adjuvant pain control.

Functional, removable braces (eg, air splints) that control inversion/ eversion, but allow dorsiflexion and plantarflexion, generally are recommended over rigid immobilization, although there is no strong data to recommend one form of immobilization over another [36]. With rigid immobilization (eg, walking boot), maximal dorsiflexion allows the least capsular distention, and thus, decreases effusion and allows for close approximation of the torn ligaments ends in grade III sprains and reduces tension on the injured ligaments in grades I and II sprains [37]. Grade III injuries may require more support than a typical air splint can offer. Remember that more extensive immobilization likely will prolong the rehabilitation period, although it may increase patient mobility earlier. Overall, early motion is an important goal in treatment. If no associated fractures are present, weight bearing as tolerated is encouraged and can be assisted temporarily with crutches or a cane. Reinforcing a normal gait pattern as soon as possible can limit stress on other tissues/joints that are proximal in the kinetic chain. The use of an assistive device for ambulation can be continued until the runner has a pain-free uncompensated gait.

Rehabilitation after an ankle sprain cannot be overemphasized. The overlying goal of any rehabilitation program is to restore normal mechanics to the ankle and improve joint stability to allow the athlete to return to safe running and decrease the risk for a recurrent sprain. Rehabilitation protocols progress in a step-wise fashion, beginning with ROM and progressing to restoring neuromuscular control, strengthening, proprioceptive training, and functional training before return to regular running.

Maintaining ROM is part of the initial management of acute ankle sprains and is the first step in rehabilitation. Passive and active assisted ROM in dorsiflexion and plantarflexion should be started as early as pain permits. Stretching with a towel for passive dorsiflexion is important to prevent Achilles tendon tightening. This can progress to standing on an incline after weight bearing is tolerated. During this early phase, low-grade mobilizations of the talocrural, subtalar, and midtarsal joints may be performed to decrease any potential restrictions, improve biomechanics, and thus, facilitate proper stretching.

Similar to vastus medialis inhibition in knee pain and serratus anterior inhibition in shoulder pain, the peroneal musculature is affected after an acute ankle sprain; thus, regaining neuromuscular control is the next step in rehabilitation [38]. Retraining the peroneals and other supporting musculature through strengthening and proprioception exercises facilitates normalizing neuromuscular control. Strength training should begin with isometrics and progress to the use of resistance bands/tubing, and finally, to closed-chain loading with toe raises and squats. The runner can progress strengthening from stress-free positions (where the ankle is neutral or in some dorsiflexion) to more stressful positions (ankle plantarflexion and inversion) and in multiple planes. More focus should be placed on the eccentric phase of contraction.

Proprioceptive training is important to recover balance and postural control, and it is hoped that it will prevent reinjury. Use of a wobble board is a common method of proprioceptive training and has demonstrated effectiveness [39]. Early on, the runner can be seated with his feet on the wobble board then progress to standing, and later, standing with closed eyes to create a further challenge for advanced proprioceptive training.

After the runner is pain-free, has full ROM, strength of more than 75% of the noninjured leg, and adequate proprioception and balance, rehabilitation that progresses to functional training can begin with the goal of increasing power and improving neuromuscular control (at the ankle and more proximally up the kinetic chain of the limb) in multiple planes of motion. Plyometrics, agility drills, and closed-chain single-leg stance exercises are part of this functional program.

Return to running is allowed when these functional exercises are performed without pain. The length of time that the athlete was in rehabilitation (and not running) will determine how quickly he or she will get back to the previous level of running. To lessen deconditioning during rehabilitation, the runner should be encouraged to stationary cycle or participate in deep-water running.

Surgical treatment rarely is the initial step, even for complete (grade III) ligament ruptures. All athletes who have an ankle sprain (grades I–III) should trial conservative treatment as discussed above. If the athlete who has a grade III tear fails this conservative approach, then consideration of surgical reconstruction is indicated after other causes for persistent pain have been evaluated fully with appropriate imaging. A delay in surgery (even years after the initial injury) does not prevent good operative results; thus, surgery should be considered only after rehabilitation has failed [40].

## Lateral soft tissue impingement

Sometimes after a severe lateral ankle sprain or repeated minor strains, scarring of the soft tissues and synovium in the area create chronic lateral ankle pain and a feeling of catching and giving-way in the ankle. Initial treatment is the same as for chronic ankle sprains. Steroid injections into the joint can relieve symptoms. If these treatments are not helpful, then surgery can be considered to remove scar tissue.

## Peroneal tendinopathy

This is a common overuse cause of lateral ankle pain and should be considered, especially if the runner has not suffered ankle sprains. Biomechanically, it is believed to be due to excessive pronation and eversion of the foot. Physical examination reveals tenderness over the tendon and pain with resisted eversion. Rehabilitation is the same as for other tendon problems: alternative training (eg, swimming, cycling) until running is asymptomatic, modalities, correction of muscular imbalances and foot biomechanics (potentially with an orthotic device), and eccentric strengthening of the involved muscles after it can be accomplished pain-free.

Subluxation of the peroneal tendon is an uncommon cause of lateral ankle pain in runners but can occur after an acute dorsiflexion-eversion stress. The peroneal retinaculum can tear, and thus allow the peroneal tendon to sublux anterior to the lateral malleolus. Treatment of an acute injury is a nonweight-bearing cast for 6 weeks. Chronic instability may be served better by surgical reconstruction because of the likelihood of recurrent subluxation.

*Sinus tarsi syndrome or subtalar ligament sprain*

The sinus tarsi is a canal that runs from the anterior inferior lateral malleolus posteromedially to just posterior to the medial malleolus. It is believed that with poor foot and ankle biomechanics (commonly excessive pronation), microtrauma can occur to this area. This injures the subtalar ligaments and connective tissue that are housed within this bony canal and cause poorly localized pain, but often just anterior to the lateral malleolus. The physical examination is nonspecific, except for pain in the area with palpation, and typically, the subtalar joint is notably stiff. It is difficult to differentiate pain that arises from the sinus tarsi from pain that is related to a lateral ligament sprain. An injection of lidocaine into the sinus tarsi that relieves symptoms may help with diagnosis. Rehabilitation is the same as for chronic ankle strains. In addition, many practitioners believe that manual mobilization of the subtalar joint is important [41].

*Osteochondral talus injuries*

The articular surface of the talus typically is disrupted by trauma and lateral lesions are associated with severe lateral ankle sprains. Typically, they are not diagnosed until further evaluation is performed in the runner who is unable to rehabilitate effectively after a lateral ankle sprain. Plain films with a mortise view of the ankle are indicated first. If negative, a bone scan that is followed by CT or MRI alone will help to demonstrate the anatomic morphology of a lesion. Conservative management, generally with nonweight-bearing immobilization, is tried first for small lesions that are still attached to the talus. Some practitioners believe that joint motion without significant loading may be better to stimulate articular cartilage healing. If the lesion is large, a loose body, or did not respond to conservative management, surgery should be considered.

*Anterior ankle pain*

The most common cause of anterior ankle pain that is seen in runners is anterior tibialis tendonitis. Physical examination reveals tenderness and swelling over the tendon, and pain with resisted dorsiflexion. Rehabilitation is the same as for other tendon injuries discussed above. Most other causes of anterior ankle pain have a traumatic etiology. Tibia–fibula syndesmosis sprains usually are not seen in isolation and generally are associated with fractures or lateral ligament injuries. Partial tears are difficult to diagnosis. Complete tears usually show up as widening of the space between the medial malleolus and talar dome and search for an associated fracture is indicated. Treatment of partial tears is similar to lateral ligament sprains, but grade III tears will need cast immobilization or surgical management.

## Medial ankle pain

A common cause of medial ankle pain in runners is posterior tibial tendonitis, which is discussed in the midfoot pain section because pain occurs over the entire course of the tendon. Other causes are tarsal tunnel syndrome (also discussed above); flexor hallucis longus tendonitis, which is more common in sprinters than in distance runners because of the forceful push off that is used during racing by sprinters; and ligamentous sprains. Medial (deltoid) ligament injuries are exceedingly less common than injury to the lateral ligaments and result from eversion stress or forced external rotation to the planted foot. Associated fractures are common. An isolated deltoid ligament injury generally is treated similarly to lateral ligament sprains, although commonly, much more time is invested before return to sport.

## Posterior ankle pain

### Achilles tendinosis

Posterior ankle pain is a common complaint in runners. The most common cause of this is Achilles tendon pain, which has an annual incidence of 7% to 9% in top level runners [42]. One study of orienteering runners found that the odds of developing Achilles problems was 10 times greater in runners than in age-adjusted controls [43]. The pathophysiology behind this disorder is not completely clear. Biopsies do not reveal inflammatory cells; therefore, the terms "tendinosis" or "tendinopathy" are used, rather than tendonitis. It is more common in older runners, and histologic studies reveal fiber degeneration and derangement of collagen fibers, so it seems to be a degenerative process. Hypoechoic regions on ultrasound that are indicative of fiber degeneration are seen in asymptomatic subjects, however, so there must be an additional unknown component to the factors that cause the development of pain. In an interesting study of elite soccer players, ultrasound imaging of asymptomatic Achilles tendons was performed at the beginning of the season. Ultrasound detected changes that are associated with tendinosis (eg, spindle-shaped thickening) in 11 of 96 asymptomatic tendons. At the end of the season, five of the subjects who had abnormal tendons (45%) had become symptomatic; only 1 of the 85 tendons that were normal at the beginning of the season developed tendinosis during the season. Four of the subjects who had abnormal tendons at the start of the season remained asymptomatic, and ultrasound at the end of the season revealed that the tendon changes had normalized. Two of the 11 subjects remained asymptomatic and still had changes on ultrasound [44]. Some scientists hypothesize that neovascularization may be the cause of pain in chronic tendonosis [45].

The history of Achilles tendinosis is similar to other tendon problems that are seen in runners; it is associated with excessive mileage, sudden increases in intensity, inadequate warm-up and stretching, and muscle imbalances. In military recruits, training in the cold is a risk factor, and is believed to be caused by increased viscosity of the mucopolysaccharides, which act as a lubricant to the paratendonous structures to allow for smooth gliding of the tendon. It is believed that this may be the mechanism behind the reason for "warming up" with light exercise and stretches to prevent tendon problems [46]. Commonly, the pain is intermittent and improves with a warm-up at first and later progresses to constant pain. Multiple physical examination signs have been described. Most commonly, the most tender area is 2 cm to 6 cm above the calcaneal insertion. One small study compared the physical examination of 10 athletes who were diagnosed with Achilles tendinosis with a control group of athletes from the same sports. The physical examination included:

Sensitivity of the tendon to palpation

Arc sign: painful or swollen area moves with dorsiflexion and plantarflexion of the foot

Royal London Hospital Test: after the most tender point to palpation is identified, the area is palpated while the patient maximally dorsiflexes and plantarflexes. Pain is decreased or disappears with maximum dorsiflexion.

The outcomes were compared with ultrasound findings of tendon disease. All three tests had relatively good specificity (0.83–0.91), meaning that they were able to identify tendons that showed no changes on ultrasound fairly well; however, the sensitivity was not as good and ranged from 0.53 to 0.58 [47].

Studies of the biomechanical faults that are associated with Achilles tendinosis found that patients are more likely to have excessive pronation, limited mobility of the subtalar joint, and limited ankle dorsiflexion range. In addition, it is believed that gastroc-soleus weakness contributes to the condition because a weak or fatigued muscle lacks energy-absorbing capacity and the muscle can no longer protect the tendon from overload and strain [48].

Although the diagnosis usually is made clinically, MRI and ultrasound are able to show tendon changes. These imaging studies can be helpful to determine if it is solely tendonapathy or if a potential tear is contributing to the symptoms. If Achilles tendon rupture is suspected, Thompson's test can be performed. The patient lies prone with the calf relaxed. The examiner squeezes the calf musculature. Normally, the foot plantarflexes. No movement is indicative of an Achilles tendon rupture.

Treatment of Achilles tendonapathy usually begins with symptom control by using ice, modifying activity, and NSAIDs, although one study showed that NSAIDs were not helpful in chronic tendinosis [48]. The use of peritendinous corticosteroid injections to treat Achilles tendon problems is controversial. Many experts believe that these should be avoided because of the risk for weakening the tendon and causing rupture; however, this has not been proven in human or animal studies. In a study of 43 patients who were followed for greater than 2 years after fluoroscopically-guided corticosteroid injections into the space surrounding the Achilles tendon, no patient suffered tendon rupture [48]. Although a third of orthopedic surgeons who were surveyed said that they use steroid injections to treat Achilles tendinosis, the efficacy of these injections is unclear. In the previously discussed study, 40% believed that the injection helped them, 53% believed that it did not change their condition, and 7% believed that they were worse [49]. A study that compared corticosteroids plus bupivicaine injection into the paratendinous sheath with bupivicaine alone found no difference between the groups at 6 weeks [50]. Injection directly into the tendon is contraindicated because this was shown to cause tissue damage in animal studies [49].

Rehabilitation focuses on correcting the biomechanical faults that were discussed above and eccentric strengthening of the gastroc-soleus complex. A study of runners who had chronic tendinosis that was severe enough to prevent running had weak calf muscle strength on the injured leg compared with the noninjured leg. All patients who were included in the study had not improved after being treated with rest from running, conventional physical therapy, shoe orthoses, and NSAIDs. Fifteen of these patients went on to have surgery, and 15 were taught eccentric calf strengthening exercises and were instructed to do them two times a day for 12 weeks. In the group that performed eccentric strengthening, all patients returned to running and believed that they were at their preinjury level by the end of the 12 weeks. Strength testing revealed that the side-to-side strength changes had resolved. The group who was waiting for surgery had no change in their symptoms during that same 12-week period. After surgery, all patients in that group also returned to running at their preinjury level, but recovery took 6 months. The investigators suggested several mechanisms by which the eccentric exercises could lead to improvement, including lengthening of the muscle tendon unit, increased muscle hypertrophy and strength, and increased tensile tendon strength [51]. Another study of eccentric calf strengthening in patients who had chronic Achilles tendinosis found that all but three of the patients improved clinically and that tendon structure normalized on ultrasound after training in 19 of 26 tendons [52].

## Other causes of posterior heel pain

Retrocalcaneal bursitis can be confused with Achilles tendinosis, but the pain is localized more inferiorly. It also can coexist with Achilles tendon problems. Posterior impingement syndrome also causes posterior heel or ankle pain. It is caused by impingement of soft tissues between the talus and the tibia in extreme foot plantarflexion. It is much more common in sprinters than in distance runners because of foot position in sprinting (ie, "toe running").

## Summary

Foot and ankle injuries are common in runners. Treatment is becoming more evidence-based for the most common of these conditions; however, further research is needed to determine the best treatments for injuries that are encountered less commonly.

## References

[1] Epperly T, Fields KB. Epidemiology of running injuries. In: O'Connor FG, Wilder RP, Nirschl R, editors. Textbook of running medicine. New York: McGraw-Hill; 2001. p. 3–9.

[2] Taunton JE, Ryan MB, Clement DB, et al. A retrospective case-control analysis of 2002 running injuries. Br J Sports Med 2002;36(2):95–101.

[3] Magee DJ. Orthopedic physical assessment. 4th edition. Philadelphia: Saunders; 2002.

[4] Birrer RB, Buzermanis S, DellaCorte MP, et al. Biomechanics of running. In: O'Connor BL, Wilder RP, Nirschl R, editors. Textbook of running medicine. New York: McGraw-Hill; 2001. p. 11–9.

[5] Geiringer SR. Foot injuries. In: Press JM, editor. Functional rehabilitation of sports and musculoskeletal injuries. Gaithersburg (MD): Aspen; 1998. p. 284–93.

[6] Agosta J. Foot pain. In: Brukner PD, Khan K, editors. Clinical sports medicine. 2nd edition. Sydney (Australia): McGraw-Hill Australia; 2001. p. 584–601.

[7] Simons SM. Foot injuries in the runner. In: O'Connor FG, Wilder RP, Nirschl R, editors. Textbook of running medicine. New York: McGraw-Hill; 2001. p. 213–26.

[8] Buchbinder R. Clinical practice. Plantar fasciitis. N Engl J Med 2004;350(21):2159–66.

[9] Riddle DL, Pulisic M, Pidcoe P, et al. Risk factors for plantar fasciitis: a matched case-control study. J Bone Joint Surg Am 2003;85-A(5):872–7.

[10] DiGiovanni BF, Nawoczenski DA, Lintal ME, et al. Tissue-specific plantar fascia-stretching exercise enhances outcomes in patients with chronic heel pain. A prospective, randomized study. J Bone Joint Surg Am 2003;85-A(7):1270–7.

[11] Kibler WB. Rehabilitation of the ankle and foot. In: Kibler WB, Herring SA, Press JM, editors. Functional rehabilitation of sports and musculoskeletal injuries. Gaithersburg (MD): Aspen; 1998. p. 273–83.

[12] Pfeffer G, Bacchetti P, Deland J, et al. Comparison of custom and prefabricated orthoses in the initial treatment of proximal plantar fasciitis. Foot Ankle Int 1999;20(4):214–21.

[13] Seligman DA, Dawson DR. Customized heel pads and soft orthotics to treat heel pain and plantar fasciitis. Arch Phys Med Rehabil 2003;84(10):1564–7.

[14] Winemiller MH, Billow RG, Laskowski ER, et al. Effect of magnetic vs sham-magnetic insoles on plantar heel pain: a randomized controlled trial. JAMA 2003;290(11):1474–8.

[15] Berlet GC, Anderson RB, Davis H, et al. A prospective trial of night splinting in the treatment of recalcitrant plantar fasciitis: the Ankle Dorsiflexion Dynasplint. Orthopedics 2002;25(11):1273–5.

[16] Rompe JD, Decking J, Schoellner C, et al. Shock wave application for chronic plantar fasciitis in running athletes. A prospective, randomized, placebo-controlled trial. Am J Sports Med 2003;31(2):268–75.

[17] Ogden JA, Alvarez RG, Levitt RL, et al. Electrohydraulic high-energy shock-wave treatment for chronic plantar fasciitis. J Bone Joint Surg Am 2004;86-A(10):2216–28.

[18] Smith J, Dahm DL. Nerve entrapments. In: O'Connor FG, Wilder RP, Nirschl R, editors. Textbook of running medicine. New York: McGraw-Hill; 2001. p. 257–72.

[19] Dumitru D. Electrodiagnostic medicine. 1st edition. Philadelphia: Hanley & Belfus; 1994.

[20] Jenkins DB, Hollinshead WH. Hollinshead's functional anatomy of the limbs and back. 6th edition. Philadelphia: Saunders; 1991.

[21] Arendt E, Agel J, Heikes C, et al. Stress injuries to bone in college athletes: a retrospective review of experience at a single institution. Am J Sports Med 2003;31(6):959–68.

[22] Nativ A. Stress fractures and bone health in track and field athletes. J Sci Med Sport 2000; 3(3):268–79.

[23] Johnson AW, Weiss CB Jr, Wheeler DL. Stress fractures of the femoral shaft in athletes–more common than expected. A new clinical test. Am J Sports Med 1994;22(2):248–56.

[24] Korpelainen R, Orava S, Karpakka J, et al. Risk factors for recurrent stress fractures in athletes. Am J Sports Med 2001;29(3):304–10.

[25] Jahnke AH, Messenger MT. Ankle injuries. In: O'Connor FG, Wilder RP, Nirschl R, editors. Textbook of running medicine. New York: McGraw-Hill; 2001. p. 199–212.

[26] Garrick JG, Requa RK. The epidemiology of foot and ankle injuries in sports. Clin Sports Med 1988;7(1):29–36.

[27] Safran MR, Benedetti RS, Bartolozzi AR III, et al. Lateral ankle sprains: a comprehensive review: part 1: etiology, pathoanatomy, histopathogenesis, and diagnosis. Med Sci Sports Exerc 1999;31(7)(Suppl):S429–37.

[28] Frost HM, Hanson CA. Technique for testing the drawer sign in the ankle. Clin Orthop 1977;123:49–51.

[29] Hollis JM, Braiser RD, Flahiff CM. Simulated lateral ankle ligamentous injury: change in ankle stability. Am J Sports Med 1993;23:672–7.

[30] van Dijk CN, Lim LS, Bossuyt PM, et al. Physical examination is sufficient for the diagnosis of sprained ankles. J Bone Joint Surg Br 1996;78(6):958–62.

[31] Stiell IG, Greenberg GH, McKnight RD, et al. Decision rules for the use of radiography in acute ankle injuries. Refinement and prospective validation. JAMA 1993;269(9):1127–32.

[32] Raatkainen T, Potkonen M, Puranen J. Arthrography, clinical examination, and stress radiographs in the diagnosis of acute injury to the lateral ligaments of the ankle. Am J Sports Med 1992;20:2–6.

[33] Labovitz JM, Schweitzer ME. Occult osseous injuries after ankle sprains: incidence, location, pattern, and age. Foot Ankle Int 1998;19(10):661–7.

[34] Knight KL. Initial care of acute injuries: the RICES technique. Cryotherapy in sport injury management. Champaign (IL): Human Kinetics; 1995.

[35] Hocutt JE Jr, Jaffe R, Rylander CR, et al. Cryotherapy in ankle sprains. Am J Sports Med 1982;10(5):316–9.

[36] Kerkhoffs GM, Rowe BH, Assendelft WJ, et al. Immobilisation and functional treatment for acute lateral ankle ligament injuries in adults. Cochrane Database Syst Rev 2002;3: CD003762.

[37] Safran MR, Zachazewski JE, Benedetti RS, et al. Lateral ankle sprains: a comprehensive review part 2: treatment and rehabilitation with an emphasis on the athlete. Med Sci Sports Exerc 1999;31(7)(Suppl):S438–47.

[38] Konradsen L, Olesen S, Hansen HM. Ankle sensorimotor control and eversion strength after acute ankle inversion injuries. Am J Sports Med 1998;26(1):72–7.

[39] Zoch C, Fialka-Moser V, Quittan M. Rehabilitation of ligamentous ankle injuries: a review of recent studies. Br J Sports Med 2003;37(4):291–5.

[40] Krips R, van Dijk CN, Halasi T, et al. Anatomical reconstruction versus tenodesis for the treatment of chronic anterolateral instability of the ankle joint: a 2- to 10-year follow-up, multicenter study. Knee Surg Sports Traumatol Arthrosc 2000;8(3):173–9.

[41] Brukner PD. Ankle Pain. In: Brukner PD, Khan K, editors. Clinical sports medicine. 2nd edition. Sydney (Australia): McGraw-Hill Australia; 2001. p. 574–83.

[42] Lysholm J, Wiklander J. Injuries in runners. Am J Sports Med 1987;15(2):168–71.

[43] Kujala UM, Sarna S, Kaprio J, et al. Heart attacks and lower-limb function in master endurance athletes. Med Sci Sports Exerc 1999;31(7):1041–6.

[44] Fredberg U, Bolvig L. Significance of ultrasonographically detected asymptomatic tendinosis in the patellar and Achilles tendons of elite soccer players: a longitudinal study. Am J Sports Med 2002;30(4):488–91.

[45] Alfredson H, Ohberg L, Forsgren S. Is vasculo-neural ingrowth the cause of pain in chronic Achilles tendinosis? An investigation using ultrasonography and colour Doppler, immunohistochemistry, and diagnostic injections. Knee Surg Sports Traumatol Arthrosc 2003;11(5):334–8.

[46] Milgrom C, Finestone A, Zin D, et al. Cold weather training: a risk factor for Achilles paratendinitis among recruits. Foot Ankle Int 2003;24(5):398–401.

[47] Maffulli N, Kenward MG, Testa V, et al. Clinical diagnosis of Achilles tendinopathy with tendinosis. Clin J Sport Med 2003;13(1):11–5.

[48] Paavola M, Kannus P, Jarvinen TA, et al. Achilles tendinopathy. J Bone Joint Surg Am 2002;84-A(11):2062–76.

[49] Gill SS, Gelbke MK, Mattson SL, et al. Fluoroscopically guided low-volume peritendinous corticosteroid injection for Achilles tendinopathy. A safety study. J Bone Joint Surg Am 2004;86-A(4):802–6.

[50] DaCruz DJ, Geeson M, Allen MJ, et al. Achilles paratendonitis: an evaluation of steroid injection. Br J Sports Med 1988;22(2):64–5.

[51] Alfredson H, Pietila T, Jonsson P, et al. Heavy-load eccentric calf muscle training for the treatment of chronic Achilles tendinosis. Am J Sports Med 1998;26(3):360–6.

[52] Ohberg L, Lorentzon R, Alfredson H. Eccentric training in patients with chronic Achilles tendinosis: normalised tendon structure and decreased thickness at follow up. Br J Sports Med 2004;38(1):8–11.

ELSEVIER
SAUNDERS

Phys Med Rehabil Clin N Am
16 (2005) 801–829

PHYSICAL MEDICINE
AND REHABILITATION
CLINICS OF
NORTH AMERICA

# Evaluation and Selection of Shoe Wear and Orthoses for the Runner

## Michael H. Yamashita, PT

*Eastside Sports Rehab, P.O. Box 6908, Bellevue, WA 98008-0908, USA*

Every athlete seeks out equipment to maximize his/her sport performance and minimize risk of injury. The two primary equipment variables in the runner's tool box are running shoes and orthoses. Runners repeatedly subject their bodies to stresses that are equal to two to three times their body weight [1,2] for a huge number of cycles each time that they participate in their sport. Few runners are structurally ideal; this results in a range of compensations that contribute to inefficiencies and, potentially, injury. The purpose of this article is to educate clinicians regarding the basic evaluation of the patient to assess appropriate shoe wear and to recognize when over-the-counter or custom orthosis intervention is necessary. To do this effectively, a basic understanding of foot and ankle mechanics is essential.

## The importance of the subtalar joint/midtarsal joint relationship

The subtalar joint (STJ) consists of the talus superiorly and the calcaneus inferiorly (Figs. 1–3). With an average axis orientation of 42° to the transverse plane and 23° to the sagittal plane, the primary component motions are eversion/abduction and inversion/adduction, with inversion/eversion occurring in a 1:1 ratio with adduction/abduction based on the average axis orientation [3–5]. The primary importance of the STJ is that its position influences midtarsal joint (MTJ) motion. The MTJ consists of the talonavicular articulation and the calcaneocuboid articulation (see Figs 2 and 3). The talonavicular joint has primary component motions of eversion and inversion (thus, the longitudinal axis), whereas the calcaneocuboid joint has primary component motions of dorsiflexion/abduction and plantar-flexion/adduction (thus, the oblique axis). Note that significant mobility in all three planes is available in the MTJ. This allows the MTJ to compensate

*E-mail address:* michaelyamashita@eastsidesportsrehab.com

1047-9651/05/$ - see front matter © 2005 Elsevier Inc. All rights reserved.
doi:10.1016/j.pmr.2005.02.006

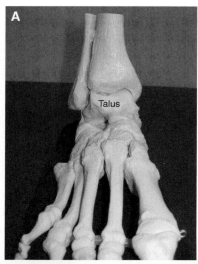

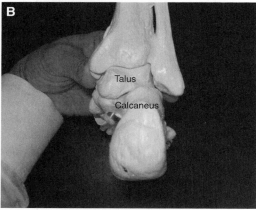

Fig. 1. (A) Anterior view of subtalar joint. (B) Posterior view of subtalar joint.

for restrictions or hypermobility in adjacent joints, which often leads to injury.

Arguably, it is the goal of the running shoe or orthosis to control the timing, rate, and excursion of STJ motion to allow the joints and muscles in the lower extremity to function in a range that is closer to that required for optimal shock absorption and force transmission. STJ position determines MTJ function because when the STJ is everted during lower extremity pronation, the MTJ axes become more parallel, and subsequently "loosen" the MTJ to provide shock absorption and to allow accommodation to variations in the running surface [6]. This should occur simultaneously through the foot, and distal to proximal in the lower limb from heelstrike

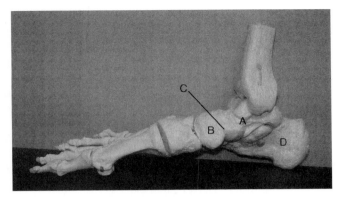

Fig. 2. Talonavicular joint. (*A*) Talus. (*B*) Navicular. (*C*) Talonavicular joint. (*D*) Calcaneus.

through midstance after which the lower extremity should begin to resupinate from proximal to distal [1]. As the STJ inverts from midstance through the propulsive phase, the MTJ axes become more perpendicular; this restricts MTJ motion and provides the lower extremity musculature with a stiff forefoot [6] with which to propel forward.

When structural deviation, muscle restriction, or weakness interrupts the normal timing, excursion, or rate of this sequence, running pathomechanics occur which negatively impact efficiency and performance, and ultimately can result in acute or chronic injury.

## Normal pronation

Pronation is a much maligned motion in the runner's vocabulary. It is, however, an essential part of the running cycle because it allows for shock absorption and accommodation for terrain when it occurs during the correct

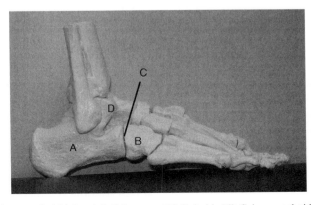

Fig. 3. Calcaneocuboid joint. (*A*) Calcaneus. (*B*) Cuboid. (*C*) Calcaneocuboid. (*D*) Talus.

phase of gait, at an appropriate rate, to the appropriate extent, and transitions to resupination at the appropriate time. Closed chain pronation of the STJ is associated distally with talar adduction and plantarflexion as well as eversion of the calcaneus which unlocks the MTJ and facilitates accommodation of the foot to the ground. Concurrent with STJ eversion, tibial internal rotation also occurs [3], which unlocks the knee and allows the quadriceps to absorb shock. As motion moves more proximal, knee flexion and valgus occur along with hip internal rotation and adduction.

**Normal supination**

Closed chain supination of the STJ locks the MTJ to provide a rigid lever for propulsion. Lower extremity motion, associated with closed chain supination, includes hip external rotation and abduction, knee extension and varus, tibial external rotation, talar abduction and dorsiflexion, and calcaneal inversion. Supination also must occur at the correct phase of gait, at the correct rate, to the appropriate extent, and with transition to pronation at the appropriate time for efficient function to occur.

**Running versus walking**

There are several obvious differences between running and walking that must be considered when making decisions about appropriate shoe wear and orthoses. The vertical ground reaction force increases to approximately three times body weight in the runner; it increases even more when running hills. There is a narrowing of the base of gait with running [7], which acts as functional tibial varum and requires increased STJ compensation. Rate and range of motion in all planes increases; however, motion in the transverse plane increases at a greater rate than motion in other planes with an obvious dominance of trunk counterrotation at greater speeds. This necessitates adequate range of motion to avoid pathologic compensations, particularly with respect to talocrural joint (TCJ) dorsiflexion, hip extension and hip internal rotation, and STJ eversion. Additionally, because of the increased rate of motion, greater eccentric control is required by the entire system. Keeping this in mind, if the STJ axis is closer to the frontal plane (high axis), as in a higher arched foot, the proportion of tibial rotation that is associated with each degree of STJ inversion/eversion becomes higher [4]. Therefore, greater effort is required to control proximal transverse plane motions that are associated with pronation.

Other differences to observe between running and walking are the decrease in vertical excursion of the head, decrease in duration of gait cycle, decrease in the ratio between time spent in stance phase versus swing phase [8], and the shift to a float phase versus double limb support. With increasing speed, location of initial contact generally shifts forward to the midfoot, or the forefoot in faster runners, which provides an argument for purposefully evaluating what features in the midfoot and forefoot of the running shoe and orthosis would be appropriate.

## Shoe anatomy

Every shoe manufacturer has its proprietary technology for cushion and motion control, but the goal and effect of each brand's combination of components is similar. The pertinent anatomy of the running shoe includes the last (refers to the shape of the shoe), which can be curved, semicurved, or straight (Fig. 4); the midsole, which can be dual density and composed of a variety of materials with varying stiffness (Fig. 5); the outsole, which, again, can be composed of a variety of materials with different durability and characteristics; the heel counter (Fig. 6), which can vary in stiffness and contributes to rearfoot control; and the upper, which can have a variety of materials that can be oriented in a manner to resist the stresses that are associated with normal or abnormal gait mechanics. The two methods by which the upper is joined to the midsole also are important. The first is slip lasting, which refers to a shoe that has a midsole that is stitched to the upper and allows the stiff foot to move more freely. The second is the board lasted shoe, which uses a firm fibrous board between the midsole and the upper and provides a more stable base for function of the flexible foot. The running shoe also can use a combination of board and slip lasting, which is referred to appropriately as a combination last.

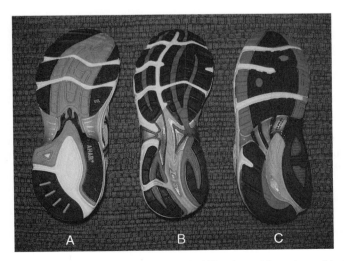

Fig. 4. Cushion shoe with curved last (Asics; *A*). Stability shoe with semicurved last (Brooks; *B*). Motion control shoe with straight last (Brooks; *C*).

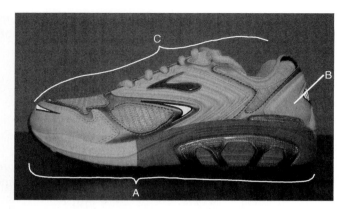

Fig. 5. Medial view of motion control shoe with dual density midsole (Brooks). (*A*) dual density midsole; (*B*) heel counter; (*C*) upper.

## Shoe types

The runner, essentially, has three broad categories of shoes from which to pick. These categories are cushion shoes, stability shoes, and motion control shoes. Features may overlap and shoe fit may vary from brand to brand, but this provides the individual runner with an excellent opportunity to find just the right shoe features and fit.

### Cushion shoes

Generally, cushion shoes are best for the patient who has an excessively supinatory gait to provide additional shock absorption, although

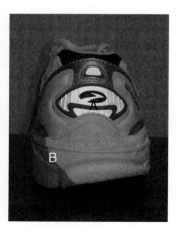

Fig. 6. Posterior view of motion control shoe heel counter (Brooks). (*A*) heel counter; (*B*) dual density midsole.

biomechanically efficient runners also can benefit from the cushioning that is afforded by this type of shoe. Typically, the shoe is built on a curved- or semicurved-shaped last and will be slip lasted or combination lasted (board-lasted rearfoot, slip-lasted forefoot) with cushioning in the midfoot and forefoot. The midsole may be broader through the forefoot and rearfoot, but narrower through the midfoot, and appears somewhat hourglass-shaped (Fig. 7A). With the absence of a dual-density midsole and with minimal additional reinforcing materials overlying the narrower midfoot region, the cushion shoe allows more pronation to occur to facilitate shock absorption. This is an obvious contrast to a motion control shoe, which is left broader through the same area to facilitate greater torsional stability (Fig. 7B). This difference becomes obvious when performing long axis and sagittal plane stability tests on the cushion shoe (Fig. 8).

One other important consideration with regard to cushion shoes is specific fit. The supinator tends to have a C-shaped foot with a high arch, a wide forefoot, and, often, a clawing of the toes which necessitates a high and wide toe box.

## Stability shoes

Stability shoes are best for the mild to moderate overpronator. Typically, they are semicurved or straight lasted and usually are combination lasted.

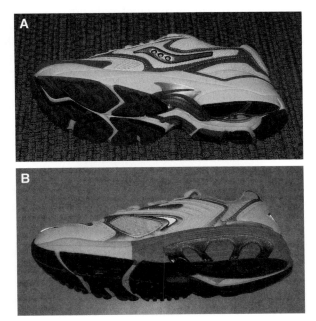

Fig. 7. (*A*) Bottom of cushion shoe with tapered midfoot shape (Saucony). (*B*) Bottom of motion control shoe with broad midfoot (Brooks).

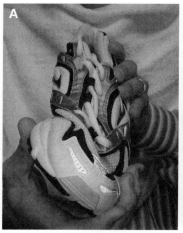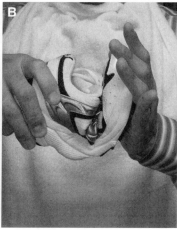

Fig. 8. (*A*) Example of deformation along the longitudinal axis allowed by cushion shoe (Brooks). (*B*) Example of sagittal plane midfoot motion allowed by the cushion shoe (Brooks).

These shoes usually provide a compromise between motion control and cushioning by using materials that assist in shock attenuation, but also incorporate some motion control feature, such as a firm heel counter; dual-density midsole; and, often, a more rigid material imbedded into the midfoot region of the midsole to facilitate greater torsional rigidity. The denser material in a dual-density midsole typically is a different color than the rest of the midsole and is present from the medial side of the rearfoot to the region just distal to the talonavicular joint, or as far forward as the region proximal to the metatarsal heads (see Fig. 5).

*Motion control shoes*

Motion control shoes are best for the moderate to severe overpronator. They incorporate all of the motion control features of the stability shoe, but also may include a reinforced heel counter; extension of the denser midsole material proximal to the metatarsal heads for greater control during the propulsive phase of gait; and a straight, board-lasted construction. When assessing the motion control shoe, the medial side of the rearfoot should be noncompressible by hand, it should not be possible to deform the shoe along the longitudinal axis when grasping the front of the shoe with one hand and the back of the shoe with the other, and the shoe should flex in the sagittal plane through the metatarsal phalangeal region, but not the midfoot (Fig. 9). Additionally, shoes should be observed from behind to confirm that the heels are vertical and that symmetry is present from side to side. This evaluation is as important in assessing an old shoe for replacement, as it is for assessing the new shoe for purchase, especially considering that it should

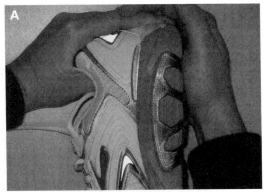

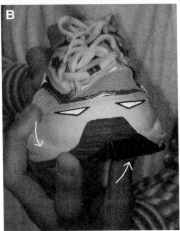

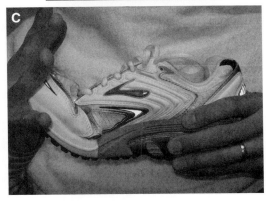

Fig. 9. (*A*) Example of medial rearfoot noncompressibility in the motion control shoe (Brooks). (*B*) Example of longitudinal axis stability associated with the motion control shoe (Brooks). (*C*) Example of sagittal plane motion occurring at the metatarsal phalangeal joints versus the midfoot in the motion control shoe (Brooks).

serve as a neutral and stable base for function of the runner who uses foot orthoses to facilitate normalization of gait mechanics.

## Anatomy of the orthosis

The biomechanical orthotic device essentially is made up of a shell, rearfoot posting, and forefoot posting (Fig. 10). Other features are used for specific issues, but these are the three essential components.

The shell is molded from a representation of the foot with the STJ in a neutral position (see section on casting technique below). The arch height of the shell can influence the rate of pronation and can provide proprioceptive feedback. In addition, the depth of the heel seat, or, conversely, the height of the shell that cups around the heel, also influences rearfoot control. The shell thickness and rigidity also can influence control or cushioning.

Rearfoot posting is a wedge that is applied to the proximal/plantar aspect of the shell to gain early control of motion or to provide cushioning at heel strike and through early stance. The goal is to influence STJ motion and position, which will influence MTJ function during the transition to midstance and propulsion. The absence of rearfoot posting, even on a neutral device, compromises rearfoot stability by allowing rocking of the shell within the shoe as a result of the rounded contour of the rearfoot portion of the shell (Fig. 11).

Forefoot posting is a wedge that is applied to the distal/plantar aspect of the shell to influence deviation from neutral alignment of the bony structures in the lower extremity. By addressing lower extremity positional deformity with a forefoot wedge, abnormal STJ compensation is prevented; this decreases compensatory pathomechanics distally and proximally. The most obvious example of this is the forefoot which is in varus when the STJ is in a neutral position. This scenario presents a situation in which the forefoot is off the ground when the STJ is in neutral and the condyles of the calcaneus are on the ground (Fig. 12A). As the foot shifts into midstance

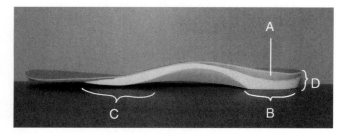

Fig. 10. Side view of orthotic. (*A*) shell; (*B*) rearfoot post; (*C*) forefoot post to sulcus; (*D*) heel seat.

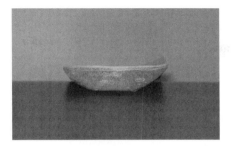

Fig. 11. Posterior view of orthotic without rearfoot posting.

and propulsion, the STJ must evert to allow the forefoot to contact the ground (Fig. 12B). This unlocks the MTJ just as it should be locking to provide a rigid lever for propulsion. This results in prolonged pronation which forces the first ray (first cuneiform and first metatarsal) into

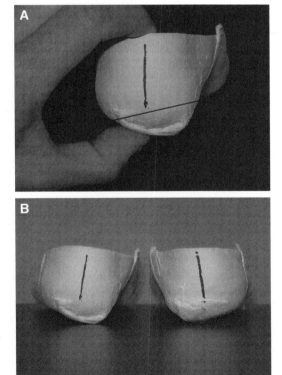

Fig. 12. Neutral STJ cast representation of forefoot varus deformity. (*A*) Neutral STJ position cast reveals forefoot varus relative to a vertical rearfoot. (*B*) Neutral casts of a patient who has forefoot varus deformity that represents STJ eversion compensation at midstance.

a dorsiflexed position and excessively loads the second metatarsal. In this situation, the forefoot post builds the ground up to the forefoot, thereby preventing the need for compensatory STJ eversion at midstance and facilitating a stable MTJ and first ray during the propulsive phase of gait.

## Types of devices

There are two types of orthotic devices. First, there is the neutral over-the-counter device which affords a nonspecific arch contour that may assist in some motion control, proprioceptive feedback, and cushioning, but fails to address positional/structural deformity and the obligatory compensations that result. In an excessively pronatory gait, the arch simply acts as a buttress to slow the compensatory pronation. In contrast, biomechanical orthotic devices address the source of the compensation and slow the rate and extent, and alter the timing of the compensation using rearfoot and forefoot posting to build the ground up to the foot. In addition, the shell acts as a support for compensatory midfoot motion. In this way, the arch contour of the custom device must only act as a secondary support, rather than a primary one, because the posting facilitates more appropriate STJ and MTJ function. This results in less compensatory inferior and medial navicular excursion (navicular drop) as well as a stable first ray in the case of early, excessive, and prolonged pronation.

Custom devices for the runner can be classified by stiffness. There are rigid, semirigid, and flexible devices. The easiest way to think about appropriate rigidity is that the rigid foot requires a more flexible device and a more flexible foot requires a more rigid device; the goal is to provide adequate stability to the flexible foot and adequate cushioning to the stiff foot.

## Importance of appropriate casting technique

Because shell contour significantly affects midfoot control, it is important to evaluate an often overlooked aspect of orthosis fabrication—the casting technique that is used by the dispensing provider. This plays a pivotal role in the ultimate comfort and function of the custom device.

A variety of techniques are used to capture the contour of the foot to fabricate custom orthotic devices. The two broad categories are weight bearing (eg, stepping into a box with compressible foam) and nonweight bearing (eg, using plaster splints to create a slipper cast of the foot). In each, the key is to capture the contour of the foot with the STJ in a neutral position. This assures that the contour of the device at midstance matches the arch contour of the patient. Obviously, the weight-bearing arch contour that is dictated by the finished device depends on the posting angles that are specified by the practitioner; they need to support a neutral STJ position at midstance to normalize gait mechanics.

Posting angles—the angles of the wedges that are applied to the rear and forefoot of the devices—are the predominant influences on STJ position in weight bearing; however, positioning the STJ in neutral while capturing the contour of the foot for orthosis fabrication is essential for comfort. If the foot is pronated, the resultant device has a lower than ideal arch contour, whereas if the foot is supinated, the arch height is higher. Less support is provided during the stance phase with the lower arch contour, and increased compression and discomfort result from a device with an excessively elevated arch contour. Capturing the pathologically compensated position of the foot in midstance, whether that tendency is toward pronation or supination, has the unfortunate consequence of a device contour that reflects and facilitates the compensated position in midstance. These errors are possible with weight-bearing and nonweight-bearing techniques, so the importance of conscientious maintenance of STJ neutral position when casting cannot be overstressed.

For this reason, it is the author's bias to use nonweight-bearing casts because it is simple to maintain STJ neutral position by palpating the head of the talus for equal medial and lateral prominence with the thumb and forefinger of one hand while applying a mild dorsiflexion force over the fourth and fifth metatarsal heads to facilitate neutral talocrural joint dorsiflexion (Fig. 13). This simulates the foot and ankle orientation in midstance with the STJ in a neutral position [9]. In contrast, it is difficult to control the forefoot with a weight-bearing casting technique, such as a foam box into which the patient steps. In this situation, the forefoot may tend to move in the direction that it moves commonly (ie, it tends to move into its typical position of compensation). This results in an inaccurate representation of the foot at midstance with the STJ in a neutral position and reduces the comfort and effectiveness of the device.

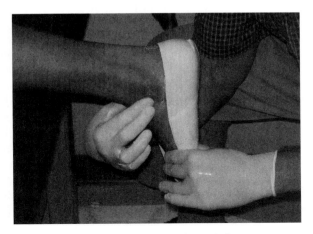

Fig. 13. Neutral STJ casting technique.

## The subjective evaluation

As with all patients, the subjective evaluation of the runner gives significant clues as to what the objective evaluation will reveal. The question of current symptoms and previous injuries gives a broader picture of the patient's history of tolerance for running as well as possible biomechanical contributing factors. Chronic symptoms, insidious onset of symptoms, and family history may point out the likelihood that structural issues contribute to running pathomechanics. In contrast, traumatic onset or first time injury may indicate injury in the presence or absence of additional biomechanical factors. Recent initiation of a running program, overtraining, road camber and surface type also can contribute to injury without a bias toward pathomechanics as a primary contributing factor.

All runners' training schedules should be scrutinized for appropriate mileage progression and appropriate rest. Intensity parameters consist of distance, speed, hills, terrain, and duration. Speed of the individual runner also should be considered because of the different predominant influences that are associated with running gait versus jogging or walking.

Additionally, timely replacement of running shoes should be stressed to maintain appropriate cushioning and control. The predominant industry recommendation has been to replace shoes approximately every 300 miles or 6 months; however, Bates and Stergiou [10] suggested that study findings are variable on this point. It is important to keep in mind that breakdown can occur more or less rapidly, depending on weight, weather conditions, terrain, and other factors.

## Objective evaluation

### Gross evaluation of gait

Initial objective evaluation should start with observation of gait while the patient is wearing shoes as well as in bare feet. Several laps up and down a long hallway should be observed, while focusing on one area of the body at a time for each lap. Watch for asymmetries, abnormal compensation, and any obvious deviation in any plane from a smooth and efficient gait. Examples of obvious deviation include excessive frontal plane motion of the trunk, excessive lumbar lordosis, asymmetrical arm swing, decreased transverse plane motion of the pelvis, obvious hip internal rotation associated with femoral anteversion, rapid and excessive internal rotation at the knees, early heel rise (typically associated with greater vertical displacement of the head), excessive out toeing/in toeing, excessive rearfoot eversion in midstance, medial/lateral heel whip, or a wide base of support. Also, listen for an abnormally loud gait, which often correlates with observation of a supinatory gait as a result of the decreased shock absorption that is afforded by this gait pattern.

These same issues should be assessed with evaluation of running gait, keeping in mind the previously outlined differences between walking and running. A treadmill and a camera with slow motion capability are helpful for breaking down running gait because of the speed at which motion occurs; however, in the context of an office visit, a few trips down the hallway should reveal the more obvious compensations. Patients who have history and evaluation findings that are suggestive of biomechanical issues, but more subtle gait deviation on visual assessment, are obvious candidates for more formal biomechanical evaluation.

This is especially important when the practitioner recognizes that some observable structural issues may or may not correlate consistently with a particular gait pattern because people have varied compensatory strategies for the same structural issues. Similarly, issues, such as a hallux valgus deformity, can stem from a wide variety of root causes. The primary issue is excessive pronation late during the propulsive phase; however, this can occur with an extremely pronatory gait, or with a supinatory gait that shifts into abrupt pronation late during the propulsive phase to influence the return of the center of gravity to a more midline position.

The specialist in biomechanical evaluation observes gait deviations and assesses the patient for specific contributory issues. Gait evaluation, in the context of this article, should alert the practitioner to any obvious gait deviations while walking and running, and should establish recognition of a tendency toward excessive pronation, supination, or a neutral gait. With experience, this also gives rise to an awareness of possible biomechanical factors which contribute to pathologic compensations.

*Simple weight-bearing tests*

Weight-bearing tests can reveal a great deal about planes of dysfunction. When asking the patient to perform a single leg squat (Fig. 14A) or to maintain single leg stance (Fig. 14B), watch for quantity of movement and quality of movement at the ankle, knee, hip, and lumbar spine. This reveals strategies to affect stability or to compensate for weakness or motion restriction. Also note any pain complaint. Typical compensation can include things, such as trunk lean and clawing of the toes. Also, watch for a tendency for the knee to shift into valgus and internal rotation, which often is concurrent with a tendency to adduct the hip in the case of an excessive pronator. Conversely, a supinator tends to lack motion into weight-bearing dorsiflexion and compensates with weight bearing back onto the heels with a concurrent forward lean of the trunk. A tendency to weight bear onto the lateral edge of the foot also is noted.

Other weight-bearing tests include single leg stance reach tests with the upper extremity or nonweight-bearing lower extremity in various directions (Fig. 15), while watching for quantity and quality of movement. Sit to stand (Fig. 16) and stand to squat tests (Fig. 17) can be performed with an eye for arch and rear foot motion and excursion. The same areas also can be observed with heel raises. Standing trunk rotation testing (Fig. 18) should

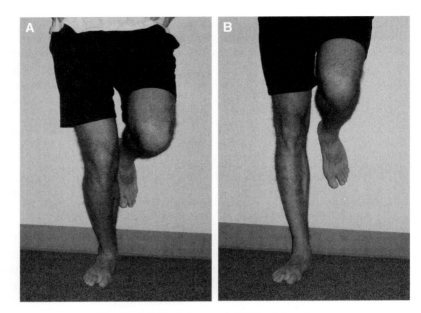

Fig. 14. (*A*) Single leg squat. (*B*) Single leg stance.

result in immediate ipsilateral supination at the foot and contralateral pronation. Although many different tests can reveal a tremendous amount of information about patient movement strategies, it is important to assess which tests provide the most pertinent information within the limited time that is available for evaluation. The most obvious strategy is to use the tests that challenge the patient to function in the most likely planes of dysfunction, based on the subjective evaluation and gait analysis.

*Standing evaluation*

The static weight-bearing examination also reveals valuable information about positional deformity, compensated positions, flexibility, and other factors that are pertinent to function. Initially, the overall structure should be observed from all sides while looking for any obvious deviations of structure in any plane. Any significant weight issue, whether due to obesity or simply a larger frame, should be noted because of the additional load that is placed on joints that are less than ideal in orientation, as well as the likelihood of more rapid breakdown of shoes. Obvious static structural associations with pronatory stress include an abducted forefoot position, significant inferior excursion of the arch in nonweight bearing versus weight bearing, an everted rearfoot position in relaxed standing (compensation for a forefoot varus deformity), tibial varum, genu varum, and genu valgum. Observable deviations that are associated with supinatory stresses include an adducted forefoot position, an inverted rearfoot position, and pes cavus.

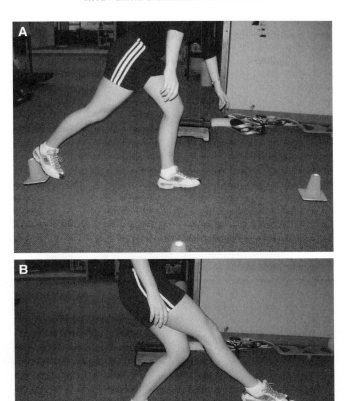

Fig. 15. (*A–E*) Single leg stance reach tests with upper and lower extremities.

One extremely important weight-bearing assessment is that of passive hallux dorsiflexion. This relates to the windlass mechanism in which the hallux undergoes passive dorsiflexion after heel off, and thus, tensions the plantar fascia, elevates the arch, inverts the calcaneus, approximates the heel to the forefoot (Fig. 19), and increases midfoot stability while decreasing tension in the ligaments of the midfoot [11]. If the STJ remains excessively pronated during late stance, midfoot ligamentous stress is increased, and hallux dorsiflexion is inhibited because the midfoot remains pronated and unstable. In this scenario, the arch fails to elevate and the peroneus longus is in a disadvantaged position, and, thus, is unable to plantarflex and stabilize the first ray to the ground [4,12,13]. Consequently,

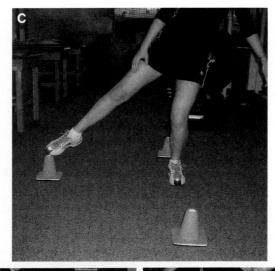

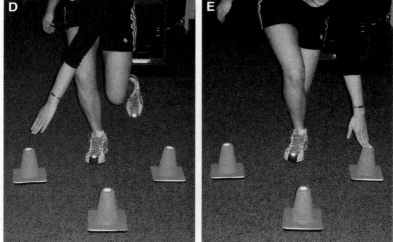

Fig. 15 (*continued*)

passive hallux dorsiflexion is unable to overcome the force that is exerted by pronatory tensioning of the plantar fascia. Michaud [14] further described the additional inability of peroneus longus to dorsiflex and evert the cuboid; this results in failure to maintain calcaneocuboid joint stability during propulsion. This illustrates the importance of assessing in nonweight-bearing and weight-bearing positions because of the compensations that may only be obvious when the foot is on the ground.

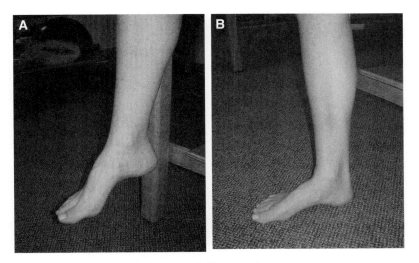

Fig. 16. (*A,B*) Sit to stand test.

## Strength tests

Standard lower extremity strength testing is an important evaluation tool. It offers information regarding deficiencies in strength that may contribute to gait pathomechanics. Conversely, gait pathomechanics can put lower extremity musculature at a disadvantage and lead to patterns of

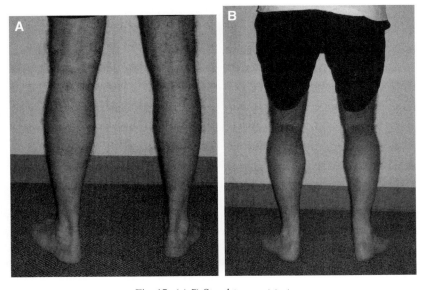

Fig. 17. (*A,B*) Stand to squat test.

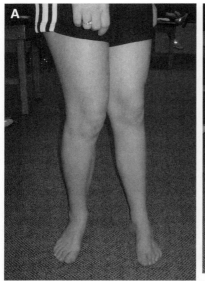
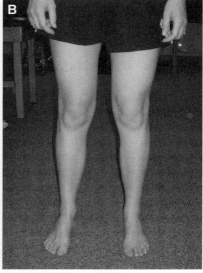
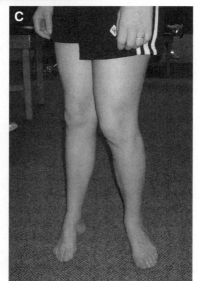

Fig. 18. (*A–C*) Standing trunk rotation test.

weakness as a consequence. Typical weakness that is associated with an excessively pronatory gait includes posterior tibialis, tensor fascia lata, and gluteus medius weakness. When observed, the question of source versus symptoms must be addressed. Did the weakness allow excessive pronation or did a structural issue lead to compensatory pronation, and thus, put these muscles at a disadvantage?

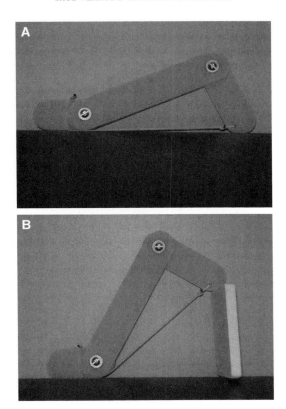

Fig. 19. (*A,B*) The windlass mechanism. Representation of arch elevation associated with passive hallux dorsiflexion.

*Flexibility tests*

Assessment of flexibility also is important in that if adequate flexibility for normal gait is not present, the body is forced to compensate (eg, if talocrural joint dorsiflexion is restricted, dorsiflexion occurs through the next joint that allows a large component motion of dorsiflexion, in this case, the oblique axis of the MTJ). The result of this compensatory gait inefficiency is a greater likelihood of injury.

*Nonweight-bearing observation*

In addition to the standard and specific functional evaluation, the nonweight-bearing examination can offer valuable information to the practitioner. The nonweight-bearing arch height can be observed and compared with that observed in weight bearing, leg length discrepancy can be assessed, and the presence of tibial and femoral torsions can be evaluated. Hallux dorsiflexion range in nonweight bearing can be assessed and compared with available range in weight bearing to determine the difference between a functional hallux limitus that is due to impairment of the windlass mechanism, and a true hallux limitus or rigidus.

When observing the plantar aspect of the foot, the presence of callus patterns should be noted, and the presence of skin folds over the plantar aspect of the feet (an indication of hypermobility) can be observed. Additionally, recognition of ankle or forefoot equinus deformity, presence or absence of a plantarflexed first ray, and forefoot varus or valgus deformity can be appreciated in prone with the STJ maintained in neutral. Assessment of these issues can help the provider to recognize the reasons behind any gait deviations or functional compensations that are observed during the weight-bearing aspects of evaluation.

## Clinical decision making

Following physical examination of the patient, the practitioner should have a basic idea of whether the patient tends toward a pronatory, supinatory, or neutral gait. In addition, recognition of some of the factors that contribute to gait deviation should be obvious. The next step is to evaluate the severity of any gait pathomechanics and decide what type of shoe should be prescribed to the patient and whether an over-the-counter or custom orthosis would be helpful.

As any experienced practitioner knows, the most important issue in treating any pathology is recognition of the source versus the symptoms. The chronicity of pathology in the runner who has biomechanical issues may point to a history of only focal symptomatic treatment. This can be effective transiently; however, without addressing the distal or proximal cause of the offending pathomechanics, recurrent injury or pain is inevitable.

## The excessive pronator

### Typical signs and symptoms

Excessive pronators present with a broad range of pathology (Box 1). They can be plagued by a variety of injuries in different areas, or experience chronic injury of the same structures. This depends on compensatory strategies and the integrity of the areas that are influenced by pronatory dysfunction at any point in time. Again, the key feature to watch for with any biomechanical issue is chronicity.

Often, the overpronator presents with early, excessive, and prolonged pronation which results in characteristic callus patterns. Ordinarily, a pinch callus over the medial hallux can be observed, which is due to the patient propelling medially over a functional hallux limitus, as well as diffuse callusing over the ball of the foot. In this situation, hallux dorsiflexion is limited because of the pathologic influence of prolonged pronation on the windlass mechanism. Additionally, when the STJ remains pronated through

---

**Box 1. Typical pathology of the overpronator**

Stress fracture
Neuroma
Hallux abducto valgus
Achilles tendonitis
Medial tibial stress syndrome
Anterior shin splints
Tarsal tunnel syndrome
Patellofemoral tracking
Patellar tendonitis
Pes anserine tendonitis/bursitis
Iliotibial band tendonitis
Sacroiliac joint pathology
Lumbar spine pathology

---

the propulsive phase of gait, the MTJ fails to lock and the peroneus longus is placed at a mechanical disadvantage. Therefore, instead of providing a plantarflexion force to maintain first ray stability for propulsion, the peroneus longus allows the ground to push the first ray up into dorsiflexion; this results in excessive loading of the other metatarsals. Consequently, callusing over the second, and sometimes, the third and fourth metatarsal heads can be observed.

Other issues that often are present include weakness of hip abductors and external rotators, as well as peroneus longus and posterior tibialis, due to the excessive loads that are placed upon these structures by this inefficient gait pattern.

*Contributing factors*

Structural issues that contribute to excessive pronation include rear foot varus deformity, forefoot varus deformity, equinus deformity, tibial or femoral torsion, and genu varus or valgus. Common contributory flexibility issues include TCJ dorsiflexion restriction and functional forefoot varus or supinatus [15,16]. The latter is a supinatory soft tissue restriction along the long axis of the MTJ which mimics the osseous forefoot varus deformity.

*Appropriate shoes/orthoses*

Depending on the severity of overpronation, stability shoes or motion control shoes are indicated. In the case of the moderate to severe overpronator, a motion control shoe is preferred. If there are not multiple areas of involvement and there is not a history of chronic injury with activity, an over-the-counter arch support may be helpful in slowing excessive midfoot compensation in the mild overpronator. If, however, the patient has experienced a variety of symptoms over the course of his/her running career, if there is an issue of chronicity, or if obvious structural issues are dictating functional compensation, a formal biomechanical evaluation should be pursued. Custom biomechanical orthoses, which are fabricated based on evaluation by a knowledgeable practitioner, should facilitate normalization of running mechanics, and thereby, assist in the resolution of the presenting issue and decrease the likelihood of injury in the future.

## The supinator

### Typical signs and symptoms

The supinator is characterized by a gait pattern that lacks shock absorption. Because the STJ remains inverted through much of the stance phase, the midfoot remains stiff and fails to assist in cushioning the impact that is associated with early stance. Typically, this is a loud gait because of the abrupt rate of loading. This gait pattern often is marked by callosities over the first and fifth metatarsal heads in the case of a forefoot valgus deformity. In this case, the forefoot sits in valgus relative to the rearfoot when the STJ is in neutral; as the forefoot loads, the first ray contacts the ground first and forces the STJ to compensate into an inverted position. Consequently, the fifth metatarsal head loads rapidly, only to shift abruptly medially as the STJ pronates to shift the center of gravity back toward midline at heel off [17]. This appears as a lateral heel whip.

The tenuous balance that is afforded by the rate and duration of lateral column loading, as well as the lack of shock absorption that is associated with this gait pattern results in the characteristic array of pathology that is noted in Box 2.

### Contributing factors

The typical supinator has a high arched foot which tends to be stiff and a forefoot valgus deformity often is present. It also is common to see a concurrent rigid plantarflexed first ray.

Another scenario is the uncompensated forefoot varus deformity in which the STJ lacks adequate eversion to compensate for the varus position of the forefoot. This foot type maintains a supinated position through stance phase with the lateral foot remaining loaded late into the propulsive phase; this creates a characteristic callus pattern along the lateral border of the foot. This necessitates an abrupt shift of the center of gravity toward midline during terminal stance which sharply loads the medial hallux.

Obviously, this tenuous balance, which is provided by weight bearing on the lateral aspect of the foot, is exacerbated in a patient who has a concurrent tibial or genu varum because of the absence of pronatory compensation in the STJ.

---

**Box 2. Typical pathology of the supinator**

Chronic ankle sprains
Sublexed peroneal tendons
Plantar fasciitis
Metatarsalgia
Stress fractures
Hammer toes
Claw toes
Haglund's deformity
Sesamoiditis
Peroneal tendonitis
Iliotibial band tendonitis
Sacroiliac joint pathology
Lumbar pathology

---

*Appropriate shoes/orthoses*

The issue with the supinator is to facilitate motion and shock attenuation. The shoe of choice, therefore, is the cushion shoe. Cushion insoles also may be helpful; however, if an obvious structural issue contributes to this gait pattern, as well as chronic pathology, a custom device is essential.

**The neutral runner**

The neutral runner tends to visit the clinic primarily as a result of trauma, inappropriate training progression, terrain issues, flexibility issues, or weakness. A stability shoe with a good combination of motion control and shock absorption is appropriate for this type of runner, but a cushion shoe also may be well-tolerated. Considerations should include mileage, terrain, and body weight when selecting more or less stable shoes on the spectrum.

**Evaluating the orthosis**

When evaluating the orthoses of a patient who arrives in the clinic for the first time, gait and quality of functional weight-bearing test performance should be observed. Next, the contour of the device should be observed and matched to the nonweight-bearing foot in a neutral STJ position. A common casting error is to capture the contour of the foot in a compensated position, which, for the overpronator, means that the device contour will be lower than the arch when assessed in the manner that was described previously. Cursory evaluation, based on the previous sections should be performed to assess the sources of weight-bearing pathomechanics, as well as to evaluate how well the devices resolve the compensatory mechanics. Full correction to an idealized gait is not necessarily the goal, but rather, gait pathomechanics should be controlled well enough to facilitate the patient's ability to function without an injury-inducing level of stress.

The combined effect of the orthosis and the shoe also needs to be considered when evaluating function. An aggressive device with motion control shoes may overcorrect a mild to moderate pronator, whereas a cushion shoe or a 2-year-old motion control shoe fails to provide an appropriate platform for comfort and function of a severe overpronator, even with appropriate orthoses.

One must recognize that orthoses influence major changes in the patient's weight-bearing environment and that they generally do not feel completely comfortable for several weeks. This emphasizes the importance of a gradual break-in process with wearing time increasing by 1 to 2 hours per day, depending on tolerance. Diffuse arch soreness and general lower extremity muscle soreness is to be expected, but joint pain in the lower extremity or spine indicates that the device may require alteration. Additionally, if the patient reports return of symptoms following a period of initial relief with the devices, undercorrection may be the problem. Referral back to the dispensing provider in each of these cases often results in a quick and effective resolution to the problem.

### Devices for the excessive pronator

When evaluating a custom device for the overpronating runner, the most obvious issue is whether the device is addressing the source of the problem. For example, if the structural issue is a forefoot varus deformity, the posting should extend to the sulcus, just beyond the metatarsal heads to control the forefoot position through the propulsive phase. If, however, the rearfoot is the sole issue, a standard length device that extends only to the region behind the metatarsal heads is adequate, as long as the rearfoot varus deformity is addressed appropriately (Fig. 20). Forefoot posting is not necessary in this circumstance, but a deep heel seat is an extremely helpful tool in the overpronator to control excessive rearfoot motion that is due to STJ compensation.

Another common issue that drives excessive pronation is one of structural deformity that is extrinsic to the foot, such as tibial varum or femoral anteversion. This type of deformity exerts influence throughout the stance phase of gait and must be addressed accordingly, with posting material used in the rearfoot and extending forward to the sulcus. A common error is to post standard length for a patient who has extrinsic issues or forefoot varus issues. This results in abrupt pronatory pathome-

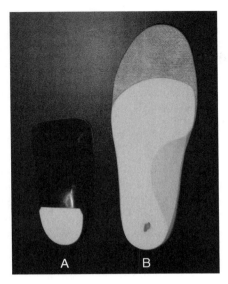

Fig. 20. (*A*) Standard length orthotic. (*B*) Orthotic posted to the sulcus.

chanics late during the propulsive phase, which force transverse plane compensation proximally. This abrupt internal rotation results in increased medial stress to the knee and lateral stress to the hip, which can affect the plantar fascia, pes anserine and trochanteric bursae, and the sacroiliac and lumbar zygapophyseal joints.

## Devices for the supinator

In the case of an uncompensated forefoot varus, a softer device with medial forefoot posting to address the deformity can help to decrease the lateral instability by distributing the forces through the entire foot versus tenuously on the lateral aspect. With the forefoot valgus, a standard length device with a few degrees of forefoot valgus posting can facilitate more normal pronation by building the ground up to the lateral side of the foot. A first ray cut-out takes away material where the first metatarsal head hits the device. This allows for more time before the first ray contacts the ground and, thereby, decreases STJ compensation into supination as forefoot loading occurs. Rearfoot control also must be considered, using a deep heel seat to control the rearfoot in preparation for forefoot loading as well.

## Summary

Many patients have been fit with orthoses and arrive to the clinic stating that their symptoms failed to resolve, or were even worse with use of the devices. Upon further questioning, they reveal that they may or may not have been evaluated thoroughly, according to the areas of evaluation that were explored in this article. Furthermore, they may have been casted in weight bearing, and often by a technician, instead of the medical provider. They usually have no awareness of having been maintained in a neutral STJ position for casting and generally remark that they were not educated at all regarding the contributory factors for their particular gait pathomechanics or pathology.

Providers who dispense custom foot orthoses include physicians, physical therapists, podiatrists, pedorthotists, and chiropractors. Because of the number of disciplines that consider foot orthoses as part of their scope of practice, the presence of a frustrating lack of uniformity with respect to knowledge base, evaluation skills, casting skills, and treatment philosophy within this population is understandable. Even the language that is used to describe positions, motions, deformity, and pathology vary based on specialty and specific training. Not surprisingly, unacceptable disparities are present, even within the same disciplines. This huge variability undermines the credibility of those practitioners who thoughtfully and deliberately fabricate devices based on sound biomechanical principles. It behooves the referring provider, as well as his/her patients, to know the background of, and the evaluation procedures that are used by, the practitioner who will be evaluating the patient for custom foot orthoses.

## References

[1] Mann RA. Biomechanics of running. In: Nicholas JA, Hershman EB, editors. The lower extremity and spine in sports medicine, vol. 1. St Louis (MO): The C.V. Mosby Company; 1986. p. 395–411.
[2] Cavanagh PR. The biomechanics of running and running shoe problems. In: Segesser B, Pforringer W, editors. The shoe in sport. Chicago: Year Book Medical Publishers, Inc.; 1989. p. 3–15.
[3] Michaud TC. Structural and functional anatomy of the foot and ankle. Foot orthoses and other forms of conservative foot care. Newton (MA): Thomas C. Michaud; 1997. p. 1–25.
[4] Novick A. Anatomy and biomechanics. In: Hunt GC, McPoil TG, editors. Physical therapy of the foot and ankle. 2nd edition (Clinics in Physical Therapy). New York: Churchill Livingstone Inc.; 1995. p. 11–46.
[5] Isman RE, Inman VT. Anthropometric studies of the human foot and ankle. Technical Report 58. San Francisco (CA): Biomechanics Laboratory, University of California, San Francisco; 1968.
[6] Mann RA. The biomechanics of running. In: Mack RP, editor. American Academy of Orthopaedic Surgeons Symposium on The Foot and Leg in Running Sports. St Louis (MO): The C.V. Mosby Co; 1982. p. 1–29.
[7] Bates BT, Stergiou N. Normal patterns of walking and running. In: Subotnick SI, editor. Sports medicine of the lower extremity. 2nd edition. New York: Churchill Livingstone; 1999. p. 157–65.
[8] Mann RA, Hagy JH. Biomechanics of walking, running, and sprinting. Am J Sports Med 1980;8(5):345–50.

[9] Fromherz WA. Examination. In: Hunt GC, McPoil TG, editors. Physical therapy of the foot and ankle. 2nd edition (Clinics in Physical Therapy). New York: Churchill Livingstone Inc.; 1995. p. 81–113.

[10] Bates BT, Stergiou N. Forces acting on the lower extremity. In: Subotnick SI, editor. Sports medicine of the lower extremity. 2nd edition. New York: Churchill Livingstone; 1999. p. 167–85.

[11] Hicks JH. The mechanics of the foot: II. J Anat 1954;88:25–31.

[12] Hunt GC, Brocato RS, Cornwall MW. Gait: foot mechanics and neurobiomechanics. In: Hunt GC, McPoil TG, editors. Physical therapy of the foot and ankle. 2nd edition (Clinics in Physical Therapy). New York: Churchill Livingstone Inc.; 1995. p. 47–80.

[13] Root ML, Orien WP, Weed JH. Normal and abnormal function of the foot. Los Angeles (CA): Clinical Biomechanics; 1977.

[14] Michaud TC. Ideal motions during the gait cycle. In: Foot orthoses and other forms of conservative foot care. Newton: Thomas C. Michaud; 1997. p. 27–56.

[15] Michaud TC. Biomechanical examination. In: Foot orthoses and other forms of conservative foot care. Newton: Thomas C. Michaud; 1997. p. 181–92.

[16] Donatelli RA. Abnormal Biomechanics. In: Donatelli RA, editor. The biomechanics of the foot and ankle. 2nd edition. Philadelphia: FA Davis Company; 1990. p. 34–72.

[17] Michaud TC. Abnormal motions during the gait cycle. In: Foot orthoses and other forms of conservative foot care. Newton: Thomas C. Michaud; 1997. p. 57–180.

ELSEVIER
SAUNDERS

Phys Med Rehabil Clin N Am
16 (2005) 831–849

PHYSICAL MEDICINE
AND REHABILITATION
CLINICS OF
NORTH AMERICA

# The Downed Runner

Paul H. Lento, MD[a,b,*], William J. Sullivan, MD[c,d]

[a]Rehabilitation Institute of Chicago Spine, Sports, and Rehabilitation Center,
1030 North Clark, Chicago, IL 60611, USA
[b]Department of Physical Medicine and Rehabilitation,
Northwestern University Feinberg School of Medicine, 345 East Superior Street,
Chicago, IL 60611, USA
[c]University of Colorado Health Sciences Center, The Spine Center at University Hospital,
PO Box 6508, MS F493, Aurora, CO 80045, USA
[d]Department of Physical Medicine and Rehabilitation,
University of Colorado School of Medicine, PO Box 6508, MS F493,
Aurora, CO 80045, USA

A downed runner who presents to the medical tent can be anxiety provoking, even for the most seasoned practitioner. Many providers do not have extensive experience with treating emergency conditions, and the perceived lack of time can cause harried decision making. Knowledge of the main life-threatening conditions that cause a runner to collapse can help with early identification and allow for specific and appropriate treatment.

This article addresses concepts that are associated with the evaluation and treatment of the downed runner. Although not intended to replace full training in Advanced Cardiac Life Support (ACLS), the first section provides a review of the initial evaluation when a downed runner presents to the medical tent. The second section summarizes the common cardiac conditions that are associated with a downed runner, including a review of the pertinent literature on sudden cardiac death and exercise-associated collapse (EAC) in runners. The third section includes a brief review of temperature regulation during exercise as it relates to hyperthermia and hypothermia. Finally, the last section covers the metabolic conditions that typically are encountered in a runner who requires medical attention, including several myths and controversies regarding fluid replacement and the causes of exercise-associated hyponatremia.

---

* Corresponding author. Rehabilitation Institute of Chicago Spine, Sports and Rehabilitation Center, 1030 North Clark Chicago, IL 60611.
*E-mail address:* plento@ric.org (P.H. Lento).

1047-9651/05/$ - see front matter © 2005 Elsevier Inc. All rights reserved.
doi:10.1016/j.pmr.2005.02.003
*pmr.theclinics.com*

## Medical support and the initial assessment of the downed runner

*Organization of the medical tent*

Medical practitioners who care for runners who present to the medical tent require appropriate equipment and assessment tools. This is especially true for the assessment of the downed runner. On-site medical facilities can become chaotic quickly, especially during races that are held on hot, humid days coupled with novice competitors and inexperienced health care providers. To ease this potentially confusing situation, a triage system should be in place in front of the medical tent to determine the nature and severity of each runner's condition as well as to provide for traffic control. The medical tent can be divided into several treatment pods with each containing a physician, a nurse, and a record-keeper. In this way, each runner is assigned a particular team to oversee and treat his/her medical condition.

A good communication system is vital to ensure prompt, efficient care. If the medical tent is receiving the downed runner from the race course, accurate information must be obtained from the local aid stations. Lines of communication also should include local hospitals in case of medical transfers. Emergent medical services (eg, ACLS-equipped ambulances) should be placed strategically at various locations on the race course to ensure adequate patient transfer to the main medical tent or hospitals, if warranted. Certain portions of the race course may be inaccessible to ambulances because of location or volume of runners (eg, bridges, parks). Alternate transportation should be considered, such as golf carts or bicycles, to expedite evacuation off the course and institute treatment.

The main medical tent should have a complete supply of equipment to treat collapsed runners properly. Box 1 lists equipment that should be available in the main medical tent. Stethoscopes, blood pressure cuffs, rectal temperature probes, and other equipment (eg, medical tables or stretchers) are an absolute requirement. By lifting the foot of the stretcher or cot up on a box or chair, the Trendelenburg position can be obtained; this often is helpful for the collapsed runner. Although scissors often are used in conjunction with bandages for treatment of wounds, they also are necessary to remove clothing for cardiac and vascular access. In addition, removing clothing will help to accelerate the cooling process in cases of heat stroke. Cooling pools and ice packs are necessary for race coverage where core body temperatures are expected to increase to greater than 40°C. Oral and IV fluids, when needed should be available, especially on hot days. Blankets and warm beverages are necessary when hypothermia is anticipated. Scales for assessment of body weight loss are helpful if prerace weight is known because weight gain may indicate fluid overload that is associated with hyponatremia [1–3]. Equipment should be available to check blood glucose and sodium concentration, because hypoglycemia and hyponatremia occur

---

**Box 1. Equipment used at medical tents that treat collapsed runners**

Stretchers
Pulse oximetry
Rectal temperature probes
Blood pressure cuff
Stethoscope
Chairs
Boxes (used to elevate foot of stretcher)
Ice bags
Cooling pools
Scissors
Wheelchairs
IV poles
Intravenous fluids and catheters
Glucose and electrolyte monitoring
Blankets
Clipboard with pens
Medical information sheets
Nebulizer treatment
Oxygen
Oral fluids (cool/warm)
Oral concentrated glucose
IV 50% Dextrose and hypertonic saline
Sodium supplement (chicken broth or pretzels)
Automated external defibrillator
Cardiac monitor
ACLS ambulance
ACLS equipment (airways/intubation tools/medications)
Scales

---

more often during long-distance races [4–7]. On-site serum sodium level can be obtained especially before instituting intravenous fluids, because intravenous fluids, other than hypertonic saline, potentially can worsen hyponatremia [6]. Finally, automatic external defibrillators should be in the medical tent with emergency transport nearby.

*Differential diagnosis of the collapsed runner*

When the downed runner presents to the medical tent, an initial assessment is performed to identify the cause of the runners' collapse. Table 1 provides a list of the more common causes of a collapsed runner.

Table 1
Causes of collapsed runner

| Mental status changes absent | Mental Status changes present |
|---|---|
| Exercise-associated collapse (misnomers include heat syncope or heat exhaustion) | Heat stroke |
| | Hypoglycemia |
| Hyponatremia | Hypothermia |
| Cardiac arrest | Hyponatremia |
| Severe muscle cramps | Cardiac arrest |
| Asthma | Anaphylaxis |
| Anaphylaxis (hymenoptera sting) | Head injury |
| Fractures, and pain-associated collapse | Asthma |

Some of these conditions are more or less likely, depending on the environmental conditions during the race (hypothermia versus heat stroke). Through the use of history; vital signs; physical examination; and occasionally, on-site electrolyte evaluation, many of these conditions can be diagnosed and treated appropriately. As in any emergent condition, airway, breathing, and circulation should be assessed first followed by obtaining accurate vital signs. Again, a calm, controlled environment can make gathering a history and vital signs much easier. For the unconscious runner, witnesses or family members can provide information that is related to the collapse and the runner's medical history. Medication use can give clues to underlying cardiac conditions, diabetes, asthma, seizure disorder, or other medical conditions. Also, some medications, such as antipsychotics, have been implicated in the development of hyponatremia [8]. It also is helpful to obtain a history of symptoms during other sporting events.

In general, any runner who presents with a change in mental status or who collapses during running should be suspected to have a more serious or severe medical problem than an athlete who collapses after completing the race [4]. Table 2 lists common clinical findings that are associated with more significant causes of an athlete's collapse [4]. One simple way to assess current mental status is to ask the runner their specific finishing time or the

Table 2
Initial assessment of collapsed runner: severity of collapse

| Stable | Severe |
|---|---|
| Collapse after run completed | Collapse during run |
| Conscious | Unconscious, or altered mental status |
| Alert | Confused, aggressive, delusional |
| Core temperature <40°C | Core temperature >41°C |
| Systolic blood pressure >100 mm Hg | Systolic blood pressure <90 mm Hg |
| Heart rate <100 beats per minute | Heart rate >50 beats per minute |
| Blood glucose 80–120 | Blood glucose <60 |
| Serum sodium 135–148 mmol/L | Serum sodium <135 mmol/L |
| Body weight loss <5% | Body weight loss >10% |
| | Body weight gain >2% |

distance where they were forced to stop. Moreover, race day clinicians should be discouraged from assuming that all collapsed runners simply are suffering from dehydration and avoid the urge to immediately begin intravenous fluids. Dehydration is believed to be an unusual cause of a runner's collapse [9,10].

Although not always true, athletes who collapse after completing a run most often experience postexercise collapse. For the purposes of this article this condition will be termed "EAC," a self-limited condition that usually is treated with elevation of the legs and time [4]. Usually, these athletes do not have significant mental status changes and respond promptly to rest in the Trendelenburg position along with oral fluids [11]. Therefore, emergency treatment can be delayed safely for 1 or 2 minutes while vital signs are obtained, rather than starting intravenous (IV) fluids automatically on every collapsed runner. The obvious exception to this would be cardiac arrest. This condition usually is identified more easily during the initial assessment and should be treated as soon as possible with ACLS and defibrillation as deemed appropriate [4]. Usually, vital signs and mental status assessment allow the clinician to formulate an initial differential diagnosis. Any athlete who has mental status changes theoretically could be experiencing a thermoregulatory problem, such as hypothermia or heat stroke, but also could be experiencing hypoglycemia, hyponatremia, or cardiorespiratory compromise [4]. For the individual who has mental status changes, initial assessment of core temperature is vital [11]. The most feasible and accepted measure of core body temperature is by way of rectal temperature [12–14]. Classically, a rectal temperature that is greater than 40.6°C is diagnostic of heat stroke, and immediate cooling is indicated [4,15]; however, rectal temperatures that do not quite meet this threshold may still represent heat stroke, particularly if the runner has mental status changes and other conditions have been ruled out. The pulse rate and blood pressure often are elevated in athletes who have heat stroke, whereas patients who have symptomatic hyponatremia typically have a normal pulse, blood pressure, and rectal temperature [5,16,17]. Runners who have arrhythmias have an irregular pulse and variable blood pressure.

Patients who have cardiorespiratory difficulties may present with a myriad of complaints and findings. Again, knowledge of the medical history is critical, particularly for runners who have asthma or cardiac conditions. Depending on the severity of the cardiopulmonary condition, mental status changes may be present and the runner will not be able to complete the race. Elevated respiratory rates with low oxygen saturation levels often are seen in runners who experience respiratory difficulties from asthma, anaphylaxis, or pulmonary edema. These athletes also may have labored breathing with wheezing. Occasionally, aerosolized β-agonists need to be instituted for the asthmatic patient. For those who have pulmonary edema, the underlying cause (eg, cardiac failure or hyponatremia) should be sought and treated [16].

Pulse rate and blood pressure may be variable in athletes who have hypoglycemia. Extreme hypoglycemia to the degree that is necessary to cause unconsciousness is rare in nondiabetic runners, but can occur occasionally in runners who participate in endurance events without adequate carbohydrate intake. This is especially true in young women who have restricted food intake as a result of eating disorders [4]. Rapid blood glucose assessment can identify hypoglycemia quickly, but other conditions need to be ruled out. Oral glucose can be ingested easily by the conscious runner; however, the unconscious or impaired runner may require IV dextrose.

Comparing prerace and postrace weight has been recommended for all ultradistance marathoners [3]. Weight loss has been reported by some to be the most accurate indicator of dehydration, yet an accurate prerace weight may be difficult to obtain [3]. Other signs of dehydration include decreased skin turgor, decreased spit production, dry mucous membranes, and persistent hypotension and tachycardia, despite Trendelenburg position. Conversely, if signs of edema, such as increased weight; hand swelling; tightness of rings, watches, or race bands; or decreased breath sounds (consistent with pulmonary edema) are detected, hyponatremia or fluid overload should be considered [4]. Medication use; estimation of food and fluid intake; urine output; and the presence of diarrhea, emesis, and other illnesses can assist in the differentiation between hyponatremia, dehydration, hypoglycemia, or other causes of collapse.

## Cardiac causes for the downed runner

Although often highly publicized immediately following a running event, the risk of sudden cardiac death in highly-trained long-distance runners is small and is estimated to be 1 in 50,000 for an intense physical activity, such as a long-distance run [18]. Other investigators estimated that 5 in 100,000 high level athletes have a serious cardiac condition that might predispose them to sudden cardiac problems; of these, 10% (1 in 200,000) may die suddenly or unexpectedly [19]. The risk in the general population is more difficult to identify. Given the increasing numbers of novice entrants into large marathons, it is more likely that the general population, rather than the elite runners, would require treatment for cardiac collapse.

Several studies have attempted to identify the incidence of cardiac death. In Rhode Island, healthy joggers had a sudden death prevalence of 1 in greater than 15,000. This doubled to 1 in 7600 if runners who had coronary artery disease were included [20]. In a Seattle study, physically active men had a risk of sudden death of 1 in 18,000 [21]. An Indiana study had a prevalence of 1 in 3600, with some discrepancy because of the difficulty with reporting or identifying the cause of death [22]. Overall, there is a much lower risk of sudden cardiac death in runners who are younger than 35 years of age [23].

## Coronary artery disease

In long-distance running, coronary artery disease is the most common cardiac condition that causing collapse. This is especially true in those who are older than 40 and includes congenital abnormalities of the coronary artery tree [19]. It was estimated that 80% of cardiac death in those who are older than 35 years of age is due to coronary artery disease [24]. Often, these athletes are perceived to be extremely fit and competitive runners, but have risk factors, including hypertension, elevated cholesterol and serum triglycerides, and a family history of early myocardial infarction or death [19]. This information is helpful to have at the time of the initial assessment of the downed runner for rapid identification of coronary artery disease as the cause of a collapse.

There have been published case series on cardiac events in runners. Noakes [25] reported on 36 cases of heart attack or sudden death in marathon runners. The mean age of these runners was 43.8 years, with an average experience in long-distance running of 6.8 years. Twenty-seven (75%) had been diagnosed with coronary artery disease, and most had premonitory symptoms that were completely ignored, by continuing to train and race through these symptoms. Half of the sudden cardiac events occurred during an event or within 24 hours of training runs or competitive events. The conclusion is that coronary artery disease does occur in marathon runners, and regular running alone is not protective against coronary artery disease, heart attack, or sudden cardiac death.

## Hypertrophic cardiomyopathy

Hypertrophic Cardiomyopathy (HC) is the leading cause of sudden cardiac death in younger athletes, with a genetic predisposition of 1 in 500 [23]. Because of abnormal muscular hypertrophy of the left ventricle, the outflow tract is obstructed. This usually is present at the subaortic septum or is due to systolic anterior motion of the mitral valve. Collapsed or near-collapsed runners may present with chest pain, palpitations, syncope, or shortness of breath. Cardiac examination findings may be difficult to assess in the medical tent, but includes a bisferiens pulse, palpable fourth heart sound, and a systolic murmur that improves with squatting [19]. ECG in a collapsed runner who has HC usually is abnormal, but nonspecific. Obviously, a chest radiograph that reveals cardiomegaly and the definitive diagnostic test of echocardiogram are not available during the initial evaluation of the downed runner [26].

## Cardiac arrhythmias

Initial abnormal cardiac rhythms, such as supraventricular tachycardia, may progress to ventricular fibrillation. Thus, automatic external defibrillators are a necessity for race coverage [19,23,27]. Other arrhythmias also may present initially as palpitations, chest pain, or syncope during or immediately after a run. Although there are benign types of sinus tachycardia with gradual onset and offset, all new arrhythmias warrant initial work-up to rule out accessory pathways (eg, Wolf-Parkinson-White syndrome) which can progress to ventricular fibrillation [28]. Also, atrial fibrillation always is abnormal, and when due to alcohol intake is referred to as "holiday heart" (rare, but not unheard of in corporate or club races) [28]. Additional work-up after the downed runner is stabilized depends on the primary cardiac diagnosis, and recommendations regarding allowing future running need to be case specific.

### Exercise-associated collapse

EAC is a common phenomenon that is a major cause of the downed runner. In ultradistance events, EAC is estimated to occur in 17% to 21% of participants; other studies reported a prevalence as high as 27% [29]. Historically, this condition was referred to as heat exhaustion when it occurred in the heat without mental status changes [30]. In reality, this is an otherwise benign postural hypotension and for nearly 60 years was believed to be due to pooling of blood in the legs associated with the cessation of exercise [31]. Unless a runner stops suddenly during a race, this typically occurs at the finish line; nearly two thirds of collapse at the finish line are due to EAC and postural hypotension [32,33]. In fact, 85% of runners who were admitted to a medical tent for collapse after finishing the marathon were reported to have EAC [32,34].

The cause of this postural hypotension or EAC probably is multifactorial. After completion of a race, there is a decrease in the muscular pumping action from the legs with a relative increased venous capacitance because of the previous athletic exertion. Additionally, regular athletic training induces adaptations to the autonomic nervous system that includes decreased vasoconstriction in response to postural hypotension [35]. The Barcroft-Edholm reflex occurs when there is a decrease in right atrial pressure. This decrease in atrial pressure which is induced by reduced blood flow (ie, blood loss) activates a reflexive paradoxic reduction in peripheral vascular resistance [36]. This reflex, combined with the increase in venous capacitance and relative decrease in muscular pumping action in the legs, results in the sensation of light-headedness; nausea; vomiting; and occasionally, mental status changes and collapse that is known as EAC.

Sweating and diarrhea that occur during the run can exacerbate the condition, but dehydration alone rarely is the cause of the collapse [4,33]. If dehydration is the cause of the downed runner, the collapse would occur during the period of physical activity in which there is maximal stress on the cardiovascular system. Runners who have EAC usually are not dehydrated [4,32,33]; fluid losses were equal in collapsed and control runners [32]. In addition, two important hormones (vasopressin and renin) that control fluid regulation also were at similar levels in collapsed and control runners [32]. Unlike runners who experience heat stroke or cardiopulmonary disorders, the overall cardiovascular status of patients who have EAC is normal in the supine position. Therefore, it is unnecessary to give these patients IV fluids; in fact, this approach could put the runner at risk for fluid overload and hyponatremia [4,32,35]. With appropriate treatment, runners who have EAC can be treated conservatively, thereby saving more intensive treatment for runners who have more severe medical conditions.

## Heat generation during running

Despite a wide range of physical activity and environmental conditions, humans must keep their body temperature between 35°C and 41°C to maintain their organ systems. Runners generate a tremendous amount of mechanical energy which is converted from chemical energy stored in ATP [4]. This conversion generates the energy that is needed to power the runner, but is incredibly inefficient [13,37]; approximately 70% of the total chemical energy that is used during muscle contraction is released as heat [4,38–40]. To prevent the body temperature from increasing to dangerous levels, runners often need to lose more than 90% of the heat that is generated. As muscles generate heat, the blood that is pumping through them is heated and then transferred throughout the body, particularly the skin. Muscles that are close to the surface also directly heat the skin by the principle of conduction. This heat is carried off by convection by circulating air currents. Any nearby object with a cooler temperature will attract the heat, whereas hotter objects, such as asphalt surfaces on hot, sunny days, will transfer additional heat to the runner's body. Sweating itself does not cause heat loss. Rather, the evaporation of sweat causes transfer of heat to the surrounding atmosphere with subsequent cooling. Windy conditions can increase heat loss, whereas humid, still conditions limit the body's ability to dissipate heat. Acclimated, fit athletes who have higher sweat rates have an easier time in dissipating generated heat. Therefore, the rate of metabolic expenditure and environmental conditions can predispose an athlete to developing heat stroke [4].

### Hyperthermia and heat stroke

Heat stroke occurs when there is a high metabolic demand with a warm environment. During a high-intensity run, the body often is in conflict between pumping blood to the muscles to satisfy metabolic demands versus shunting blood to the skin to assist in heat loss. The metabolic demands of muscles are favored. When athletes are running at a fast pace for a short duration (10–15 km), there is marked limitation of blood flow to the skin. Therefore, the runner depends on favorable environmental conditions to maintain temperature balance [41]. High heat and humidity further limit the skin's ability to dissipate heat. It is under these conditions that heat stroke is most likely to occur [4].

The thalamus reacts to an increase in core temperature by increasing the sweat response and the respiratory rate [15]. With heat stroke, there is a thermoregulatory failure with an exaggerated acute phase response to heat and alteration of otherwise protective heat shock proteins [15]. It has been postulated that those who are prone to heat stroke have a genetic predisposition, similar to the genetic condition of malignant hyperthermia. In this way, some cases of heat stroke are described as exercise-induced malignant hyperthermia [4,42].

Several risk factors are associated with hyperthermia. These include obesity; poor training methods (including not acclimatizing to running in heat); running too fast; wearing clothing with higher insulating capacity; races run during the heat of the day with poor shading; recent febrile illness; and certain medications, including diuretics, ephedra, and some antidepressants (which may inhibit sweat response) [15,43]. Often, runners ignore warning signs, and they do not recognize previous episodes as a possible indication of genetic predisposition. Prevention of hyperthermia can be achieved with proper training, avoiding running when ill, running at a cooler time of day, recognizing early warning signs, using frequent cooling stations, and ingesting fluids ad libitum.

Heat stroke is a true medical emergency which is classified as a systemic inflammatory response with an internal body temperature of greater than 41°C [4,15]. With this uncontrolled increase in core body temperature, there are associated mental status changes, including anxiety; confusion; bizarre behavior; loss of coordination; hallucinations; agitation; seizures; and often, coma. If untreated, varying degrees of multiple system organ failure ensue. These include acute renal and liver failure, respiratory insufficiency, and others. Animal studies suggested that reduced cardiac functional reserve is due to heat stroke; large IV infusions in patients who had heat stroke have been known to produce heart failure [45]. Because heat stroke is not caused solely by dehydration, the tendency to begin rapid infusion of large-volume IV fluids immediately should be tempered [46,47].

The primary treatment for heat stroke is decrease of body temperature to less than 38°C as quickly as possible. Although there had been suggestions to use wet towels, cooling fans, or ice packs, multiple studies have shown that the best method of cooling is to apply iced water directly to the skin. This is performed by placing the runner's torso in a small bath of iced water with the legs and arms hanging over the edge of the bath [48–50]. Similar methods reportedly have been used since 1917 [51]. One caveat is that rates of cooling can approach 1°C per minute [49]. Because rectal temperature lags behind core (esophageal) temperature during rapid cooling, the ice water bath should be terminated before rectal temperature becomes normal. When the temperature decreases to approximately 39°C, the runner usually regains consciousness. At this time, correction of hypoglycemia and dehydration can take place; however, IV fluids never should be the sole treatment. In addition, care should be taken to avoid fluid overload by limiting IV fluids to 1 L to 2 L [10,52]. Although some investigators have suggested managing victims of heat stroke at the race and releasing them after 60 to 90 minutes, it probably is prudent to have runners evaluated at hospital to evaluate for organ abnormalities [4]. This is necessary if the runner develops complications or does not regain consciousness quickly. Because the temperature can increase again as a result of the continued metabolic processes, observation and assessment of elevated temperature and organ failure should continue during transport to a medical facility [4].

## Other heat-related conditions

Historically, the terms "heat exhaustion," "heat syncope," and "heat prostration" were used to describe collapse that occurred at the end of an event as a result of postural hypotension in persons who were exercising on a hot day [53]. These terms should not be confused with collapse that is due to abnormal temperature regulation nor considered to be a mild form of heat stroke. In these individuals, rectal temperatures are not elevated [32,35]. There is no evidence that these runners will develop heat stroke if left to their own devices, nor is there evidence that these individuals are more dehydrated [4]. These conditions, as well as heat cramps, also have been described in coal miners, firefighters, and others [6]. A review of the early literature of heat cramps suggests that this condition is due to the loss of salt and water from the body with replacement only with water. The decrease of sodium and chloride to a critical level may lead to muscle cramps in the working individuals and athletes [6].

## Hypothermia

Hypothermia, conversely, is caused by an ambient temperature which allows the internal temperature to decrease to less than 35°C. This usually is due to running in lower temperature conditions with insufficient insulating clothing. Many inexperienced runners wear mesh tank tops and shorts. Combining this with slower running rates—during which much less muscular heat is generated—and inclement weather conditions (eg, cold temperatures, rain, wind) is a setup for hypothermia. A study of marathon runners in Minnesota found that three times as many participants required treatment for hypothermia as for heat stroke [44]. Prevention is primarily dependent on the individual runner having proper clothing. Treatment requires the ability of medical personnel to provide adequate warming.

## Hyponatremia

Exercise-associated hyponatremia, defined as serum sodium of less than 135 mmol/L, has become a recognized cause of the downed runner. Frizzell et al [54] and Noakes et al [6,55] were among the first to describe cases of this disorder in ultradistance athletes, whereas Nelson et al [56] and Young and Rinaldo [16] described the first cases in marathoners. Because of enhanced awareness, this condition is becoming recognized increasingly [57]. Hiller and O'Toole [58] reported that 25% of noncollapsed triathletes may have hyponatremia. Symptomatic hyponatremia occurs in only 0.3% of marathon runners [5], but Noakes et al [59] estimated that 9% of collapsed ultra-endurance athletes may be suffering from this potentially lethal condition.

Runners who have hyponatremia may present with a myriad of complaints. More commonly these symptoms include nausea, vomiting, abdominal bloating, headache, incoordination, fasciculations, lightheaded-ness, coughing, and seizures [3,4,6,17]. Because of peripheral edema, patients state that rings or watches feel tight. If this condition goes unrecognized or if it is treated inappropriately with IV fluids, a further decrease in serum sodium results. Hyponatremia may lead to pulmonary and cerebral edema, coma, and eventual death. Clinical signs may include confusion, wheezing, peripheral edema, and mental status changes [4]. As opposed to heat stroke, which also has mental status changes, runners who have hyponatremia typically have a normal pulse and blood pressure [5,16,17].

*Theories about the causes of exercise-associated hyponatremia*

The most commonly accepted reason for exercise-associated hyponatremia is excessive volitional fluid intake [20,60]. Evidence for this theory include a decrease in hematocrit, weight gain, and excessive diuresis in patients with hyponatremia. However, Hiller [61] cited that the problem is not with excessive fluid consumption, but rather the excessive loss of sodium. He suggested that replacing only the fluid and not the sodium chloride losses during prolonged exercise was responsible for hyponatremia. A study by Barr et al [62] refuted this. In this study, exercising athletes ingested water or low concentration salt solutions that replaced the fluid loss from sweat. Despite large unreplaced sodium chloride losses from sweat, serum sodium concentration decreased only slightly in the groups that ingested water or salt solution. In the groups who did not ingest any fluid, serum sodium concentrations increased; this suggested that dehydration actually provided protection against the development of hyponatremia. Irving et al [60] also showed that sodium losses alone did not produce low serum sodium. In this study, hyponatremic subjects did not lose larger amounts of sodium in sweat than normonatremic runners. From these studies, it is highly unlikely that sodium loss alone or in conjunction with fluid replacement is responsible for the development of low serum sodium levels in distance runners.

Relative fluid overload from abnormal renal function seems to be another plausible explanation for the development of this inscrutable disorder. Irving et al [60] hospitalized eight runners who had severe hyponatremia (serum sodium <130 mmol/L) and studied their renal function, fluid, and electrolyte balance over a 12- to 36-hour period. During this period, all of the symptomatic subjects' sodium concentrations normalized after large volumes of urine were excreted. Most hyponatremic runners lose weight upon recovery [20]. Because of this normal urinary output, it was concluded that renal function is normal in hyponatremic individuals [60].

Other studies, however, suggested that renal dysfunction occurs in exercise-associated hyponatremia. For example, a case series showed an inappropriate elevation of antidiuretic hormone in hyponatremic athletes [63]. Conversely, Speedy et al [20] demonstrated normal aldosterone and decreased arginine vasopressin levels in hyponatremic ultradistance triathletes compared with controls. This seems to dispel the theory that elevated renal hormones and an impaired renal response are responsible for the exercise-related hyponatremia.

Despite these arguments, others believe that a renal mechanism contributes to the development of hyponatremia. Montain et al [64] proposed that intense exercise increases sympathetic activity, and thus, produces a reduction in renal blood flow and glomerular filtration rate. As one exercises, less urine is produced, despite fluid intake. The combination of these factors eventually leads to a state of positive fluid balance and a dilutional hyponatremia develops; however, this theory seems to be counterintuitive because the sodium concentration, rather than extracellular fluid volume, is the regulated variable in the normal healthy state [65,66].

Some investigators suggested that exercise-related hyponatremia results from a combination of fluid retention within the gastrointestinal (GI) system and subsequent movement of sodium into third space [6,64]. It has been estimated that 1.8 L of fluid would need to be unabsorbed from the gut to induce this third-space effect. Although it seems unreasonable to think that so much fluid could remain in the gut during a race, many studies showed that the intestinal absorption of water is reduced during exercise. One study showed that only 37% of fluid perfuses across the duodenum and jejunum during exercise when fluids are ingested at rates of 900 mL/h [67]. Over the course of a 5- to 6-hour race, hypotonic fluids may accumulate within the GI tract. If carbohydrates are ingested as well, further fluid accumulation occurs. It was shown that when carbohydrates are present in the GI tract, the amount of fluid absorbed is reduced [68]. When this large amount of low sodium–containing fluid is present in the GI tract, sodium is secreted down its concentration gradient and into this third space. Animal studies showed that when a 5% carbohydrate solution was injected into the peritoneum, sodium was secreted into this third space and produced biochemical features that were indistinguishable from those that are reported in runners who have hyponatremia [69]. Therefore, the presence of a large amount of low-sodium, high-carbohydrate–containing solution in the gut will induce secretion of sodium down its concentration gradient into this third space and induce a state of hyponatremia.

The retention of this fluid within the GI tract may help to explain why some athletes who have hyponatremia often complain of nausea, vomiting, and abdominal bloating [5,17]. One also would assume that diarrhea would occur frequently, but clinically, this is not reported commonly in those who have hyponatremia [64]. Support for the theory that fluid accumulation in the GI tract and the subsequent secretion of sodium into this third space has not been substantial [70].

*Risk factors*

Certain risk factors may predispose athletes for the development of hyponatremia. The most important of these seems to be the excessive ingestion of fluids during a run. Slower runners spend more time on the course and tend to ingest excessive amounts of fluids for fear of becoming dehydrated. When symptoms of confusion, lightheadedness, and fatigue set in, they mistakenly confuse these symptoms for dehydration and, to their detriment, drink more. This has prompted some investigators to suggest that water stations of a marathon be closed at 4 hours to prevent cases of hyponatremia that are due to excessive fluid intake [71]. Additionally, it is recommended that athletes measure their typical fluid losses by measuring weight before and after a long run [71]. On race day, runners should not ingest fluid amounts that exceed the amount of fluid loss that is due to sweating. Some have suggested that runners even may be safer being underhydrated; however, this remains controversial [4,10].

Apparently women, particularly of smaller build, have a higher predilection for the development of this disorder. At the 2000 Houston Marathon, a disproportionate number of female athletes who had hyponatremia presented to the medical tent [5]. In San Diego, 23 of 26 marathoners who were sent to hospitals for hyponatremia were female [72]. Three of these women seized and spent time in the ICU. Although the reason for this is unknown, it is possible that women may ingest fluids at rates that are recommended for larger male athletes who may have higher fluid requirements and run at faster rates.

Certain medications have been implied as risk factors for the development of exercise-associated hyponatremia. Antipsychotics are known to be associated with low serum sodium levels [73]. Some investigators suggested that nonsteroidal anti-inflammatory drugs (NSAIDs) are associated with this disorder as well [57,74]. Although this has not been proven, there may be an association between NSAIDs and renal blood flow and sodium regulation.

Although most cases of exercise-related hyponatremia are caused by fluid overload, some cases may be due to subclinical cases of cystic fibrosis (CF). Patients who have CF have abnormally high concentrations of sodium chloride in sweat and typically have respiratory and pulmonary problems with a shorter than normal life span. There are more than 800 variants of the CF gene, most of which have no clinical significance. Montain et al [64], citing cases in the military, proposed that some athletes, when participating in endurance events, may lose a significant amount of sodium in sweat because of the presence of one of these CF variants. This theory has yet to be proven, but may be considered in cases of hyponatremia in which there is no identifiable risk factor, such as overhydration.

## Prevention and treatment of hyponatremia

Because hyponatremia can be a life-threatening condition, it is important to know how to treat and prevent it. Most importantly, the lay public and clinicians who care for endurance athletes must be educated regarding the potential hazards of excessive fluid ingestion. Being well-acclimatized, identifying early warning signs, and avoiding overhydration are keys to prevention. In general, athletes never should drink more than they sweat [4,71]. One practical way to estimate sweat losses is to weigh oneself naked prior to a run, then redress and run for 1 hour at a pace that is anticipated on race day. At the completion of this run, dry off and reweigh without clothes. For every pound lost, one should drink a pint of fluid (preferably sports drink, rather than water) per hour on the day of the actual race [71]. The addition of salt (eg, pretzels, soup) toward the end of the run also may be helpful. It also seems prudent to avoid medications, when medically appropriate, that may be associated with the development of this condition.

The most important factor about the treatment of hyponatremia is making the correct diagnosis. It has become common practice for clinicians who care for collapsed runners to assume that all athletes are suffering from dehydration and should be treated with aggressive IV fluids. Noakes [10,52] has urged against this practice. In his opinion, it rarely is necessary to treat a collapsed athlete with IV fluids because most runners, if not all, are not suffering from dehydration. Instead of the injudicious use of IV fluids, Noakes has pushed for the "masterful inactivity" approach for many downed runners. Many runners, especially those who collapse after completion of a run, respond to the Trendelenburg position. If mental status changes are present or if the runner does not respond to this position, then hyponatremia or another diagnosis needs to be considered (Fig. 1). If one indiscriminately used IV fluids to treat all collapsed athletes, and hyponatremia is present, the condition may worsen to the point of producing pulmonary and cerebral edema, and potentially, death [4,52].

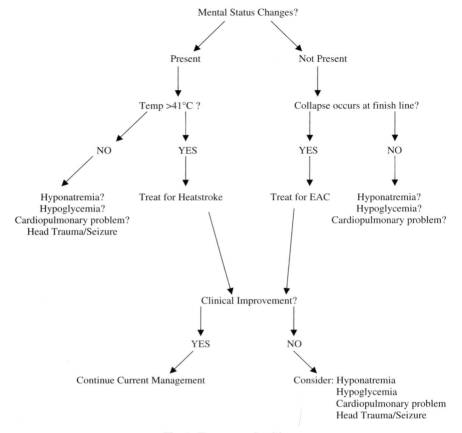

Fig. 1. Treatment algorithm.

If hyponatremia is identified and the patient is only mildly symptomatic, an attempt at treatment in the medical tent with pretzels or soup may be considered. If the runner does not respond or if s/he has a more severe presentation, transportation to the hospital is recommended. Some cases may need monitoring, and possibly, treatment with diuretics or IV hypertonic saline; however, spontaneous diuresis often corrects this electrolyte abnormality [16,57].

**Summary**

Race coverage can be a rewarding experience for the sports medicine clinician. Several conditions are likely to present to the medical tent, and accurate diagnosis is critical to proper treatment. An algorithm approach as outlined in this article can provide a starting point for the assessment of the downed runner. Recognition of the primary causes for collapse can help to instigate the correct treatment approach. A proper history and physical examination often can help to differentiate significant cardiac events from the more innocuous EAC. Furthermore, avoiding immediate IV fluids in the downed runner is prudent, at least until an appropriate diagnosis is made. This will help to prevent iatrogenic hyponatremia. In sum, proper preparation and knowledge of the ailments that affect long distance runners will help to maintain an effective medical tent on race day.

## References

[1] Speedy DB, Campbell R, Mulligan G, et al. Weight changes and serum sodium concentrations after an ultradistance multisport triathlon. Clin J Sport Med 1997; 7(2):100–3.

[2] Speedy DB, Faris JG, Hamlin M, et al. Hyponatremia and weight changes in an ultradistance triathlon. Clin J Sport Med 1997;7(3):180–4.

[3] Speedy DB, Noakes TD, Rogers IR, et al. Hyponatremia in ultradistance triathletes. Med Sci Sports Exerc 1999;31(6):809–15.

[4] Noakes T. Temperature regulation during exercise. In: Noakes T, editor. Lore of running. 4th edition. Cape Town (South Africa): Oxford University Press Southern Africa; 2003. p. 175–255.

[5] Hew TD, Chorley JN, Cianca JC, et al. The incidence, risk factors, and clinical manifestations of hyponatremia in marathon runners. Clin J Sport Med 2003;13(1):41–7.

[6] Noakes TD. The hyponatremia of exercise. Int J Sport Nutr 1992;2(3):205–28.

[7] Barr SI, Costill DL. Water: can the endurance athlete get too much of a good thing? J Am Diet Assoc 1989;89:1629–32.

[8] Siegel AJ, Baldessarini RJ, Klepser MB, et al. Primary and drug-induced disorders of water homeostasis in psychiatric patients: principles of diagnosis and management. Harv Rev Psychiatry 1998;6(4):190–200.

[9] Noakes T. Dehydration during exercise: what are the real dangers? Clin J Sports Med 1995;5: 123–8.

[10] Noakes TD. Hyponatremia or hype? Phys Sportsmed 2001;29:27–32.

[11] Roberts W. Exercise-associated collapse in endurance events: a classification system. Phys Sportsmed 1989;17(5):49–57.

[12] Armstrong LE, Epstein Y, Greenleaf JE, et al. American College of Sports Medicine position stand. Heat and cold illnesses during distance running. Med Sci Sports Exerc 1996;28(12): i–x.

[13] Cheuvront SN, Haymes EM. Thermoregulation and marathon running: biological and environmental influences. Sports Med 2001;31(10):743–62.

[14] Roberts W. Assessing core temperature in collapsed athletes: what's the best method? Phys Sportsmed 1994;22(8):49–55.

[15] Pluth Yeo T. Heat stroke: a comprehensive review. AACN Clin Issues 2004;15(2):280–93.

[16] Young MSF, Rinaldo J. Delirium and pulmonary edema after completing a marathon. Am Rev Respir Dis 1987;136:737–9.

[17] Lento PH, Akuthota V. Confusion in a marathoner. Med Sci Sports Exerc 2002;34(5):S219.

[18] Maron BJ, Poliac LC, Roberts WO. Risk for sudden cardiac death associated with marathon running. J Am Coll Cardiol 1996;28(2):428–31.

[19] Hillis WS, McIntyre PD, Maclean J, et al. ABC of sports medicine. Sudden death in sport. BMJ 1994;309:657–60.

[20] Speedy DB, Rogers IR, Noakes TD, et al. Exercise-induced hyponatremia in ultradistance triathletes is caused by inappropriate fluid retention. Clin J Sport Med 2000;10(4):272–8.

[21] Siscovick DS, Weiss NS, Fletcher RH, et al. The incidence of primary cardiac arrest during vigorous exercise. NEJM 1984;311(14):874–7.

[22] Waller BF, Hawley DA, Clark MA, et al. Incidence of sudden athletic deaths between 1985 and 1990 in Marion County, Indiana. Clin Cardiol 1992;15(11):851–8.

[23] Hosey RG, Armsey TD. Sudden cardiac death. Clin Sports Med 2003;22(1):51–66.

[24] Maron BJ, Epstein SE, Roberts WC. Causes of sudden death in competitive athletes. J Am Coll Cardiol 1986;7(1):204–14.

[25] Noakes TD. Heart disease in marathon runners: a review. Med Sci Sports Exerc 1987; 19(3):187–94.

[26] Frazier JE II. Acute cardiac emergencies in the injured athlete. Clin Sports Med 1989; 8(1):81–90.

[27] Dent JM. Congenital heart disease and exercise. Clin Sports Med 2003;22(1):81–99.

[28] Mounsey JP, Ferguson JD. The assessment and management of arrhythmias and syncope in the athlete. Clin Sports Med 2003;22(1):67–79.

[29] Speedy DB, Thompson JM, Rodgers I, et al. Oral salt supplementation during ultradistance exercise. Clin J Sport Med 2002;12(5):279–84.

[30] Adolph E. Physiological fitness for the desert. Fed Proc 1943;2:158–64.

[31] Eichna LWHS, Bean WB. Post-exertional orthostatic hypotension. Am J Med Sci 1947; 213(6):641–54.

[32] Holtzhausen LM, Noakes TD, Kroning B, et al. Clinical and biochemical characteristics of collapsed ultra-marathon runners. Med Sci Sports Exerc 1994;26(9):1095–101.

[33] Speedy DB, Noakes TD, Holtzhausen LM. Exercise-associated collapse: postural hypotension, or something deadlier? Phys Sportsmed 2003;31(3):23–9.

[34] Holtzhausen LM, Noakes TD. The prevalence and significance of post-exercise (postural) hypotension in ultramarathon runners. Med Sci Sports Exerc 1995;27(12):1595–601.

[35] Holtzhausen LM, Noakes TD. Collapsed ultraendurance athlete: proposed mechanisms and an approach to management. Clin J Sport Med 1997;7(4):292–301.

[36] Noakes T. The forgotten Barcroft/Edholm reflex: potential role in exercise associated collapse. Br J Sports Med 2003;37:277–8.

[37] Kushmerick MJ, Larson RE, Davies RE. The chemical energetics of muscle contraction. I. Activation heat, heat of shortening and ATP utilization for activation-relaxation processes. Biol Sci 1969;174(136):293–313.

[38] Magaria RCP, Aghems P. Energy cost of running. J Appl Phys 1963;18:367–70.

[39] Gonzalez-Alonso J, Calbet JA, Nielsen B. Metabolic and thermodynamic responses to dehydration-induced reductions in muscle blood flow in exercising humans. J Physiol 1999;520:577–89.

[40] Gonzalez-Alonso J, Quistorff B, Krustrup P, et al. Heat production in human skeletal muscle at the onset of intense dynamic exercise. J Physiol 2000;524:603–15.

[41] Pugh L. The gooseflesh syndrome (acute anhidrotic heat exhaustion) in long distance runners. Br J Phys Educ 1972;3:IX–XII.

[42] Simon HB. Hyperthermia. NEJM 1993;329:483.

[43] Noakes TD, Adams BA, Myburgh KH, et al. The danger of an inadequate water intake during prolonged exercise. A novel concept re-visited. Eur J Appl Phys 1988;57:210–9.

[44] Roberts WO. A 12-yr profile of medical injury and illness for the Twin Cities Marathon. Med Sci Sports Exerc 2000;32(9):1549–55.

[45] Daily WM, Harrison TR. A study of the mechanism and treatment of experimental heat pyrexia. Am J Med Sci 1948;215:42–55.

[46] Noakes TD. 1996 J.B. Wolffe memorial lecture. Challenging beliefs: ex Africa semper aliquid novi. Med Sci Sports Exerc 1997;29:571–90.

[47] Noakes TD. Physiological models to understand exercise fatigue and the adaptations that predict or enhance athletic performance. Scand J Med Sci Sports 2000;10(3):123–45.

[48] Costrini A. Emergency treatment of exertional heatstroke and comparison of whole body cooling techniques. Med Sci Sports Exerc 1990;22:15–8.

[49] Armstrong LE, Crago AE, Adams R, et al. Whole-body cooling of hyperthermic runners: comparison of two field therapies. Am J Emerg Med 1996;14:355–8.

[50] Kielblock AJ, vanRensberg JP, Franz RM. Body cooling method as a method for reducing hyperthermia. South Afr Med J 1986;69:378–80.

[51] Gauss HM, Meyer KA. Heatstroke: report of one-hundred and fifty-eight cases from Cook County Hospital. Am Jrl Med Sci 1917;154:554–64.

[52] Noakes T. Hyponatremia in distance athletes: pulling the IV on the "dehydration myth". Phys Sportsmed 2000;28:71–6.

[53] Noakes T. Fluid and electrolyte disturbances in heat illness. Int J Sports Med 1998;19:S146–9.

[54] Frizzell RT, Lang GH, Lowance DC, et al. Hyponatremia and ultramarathon running. JAMA 1986;255(6):772–4.

[55] Noakes TD, Goodwin N, Rayner BL, et al. Water intoxication: a possible complication during endurance exercise. Med Sci Sports Exerc 1985;17(3):370–5.

[56] Nelson PB, Robinson AG, Kapoor W, Rinaldo J. Hyponatremia in a marathoner. Phys Sportsmed 1988;16:78–88.

[57] Ayus JC, Varon J, Arieff AI. Hyponatremia, cerebral edema, and noncardiogenic pulmonary edema in marathon runners. Ann Intern Med 2000;132:711–4.

[58] Hiller W, O'Toole F. Plasma electrolyte and glucose changes during the Hawaiian Ironman Triathlon. Med Sci Sports Exerc 1985;17:219.

[59] Noakes TD, Norman RJ, Buck RH, et al. The incidence of hyponatremia during prolonged ultraendurance exercise. Med Sci Sports Exerc 1990;22(2):165–70.

[60] Irving RA, Noakes TD, Buck R, et al. Evaluation of renal function and fluid homeostasis during recovery from exercise-induced hyponatremia. J Appl Physiol 1991;70(1):342–8.

[61] Hiller WD. Dehydration and hyponatremia during triathlons. Med Sci Sports Exerc 1989; 21(Suppl 5):S219–21.

[62] Barr SI, Costill DL, Fink WJ. Fluid replacement during prolonged exercise: effects of water, saline, or no fluid. Med Sci Sports Exerc 1991;23(7):811–7.

[63] Zelingher J, Putterman C, Ilan Y, et al. Case series: hyponatremia associated with moderate exercise. Am J Med Sci 1996;311(2):86–91.

[64] Montain SJ, Sawka MN, Wenger CB. Hyponatremia associated with exercise: risk factors and pathogenesis. Exerc Sport Sci Rev 2001;29(3):113–7.

[65] Nose H, Mack GW, Shi XR, et al. Role of osmolality and plasma volume during rehydration in humans. J Appl Physiol 1988;65:325–31.

[66] Nose H, Mack GW, Shi XR, et al. Shift in body fluid compartments after dehydration in humans. J Appl Phys 1988;65:318–24.

[67] Gisolfi CV, Spranger KJ, Summers RW, et al. Effects of cycle exercise on intestinal absorption in humans. J Appl Physiol 1991;71:2518–27.

[68] Williams JH, Maher M, Jacobson ED. Relationship of mesenteric blood flow to intestinal absorption of carbohydrates. Jrl Lab Clin Med 1976;63:853–63.

[69] Danowski T, Winkler AW, Elkinton JR. The treatment of shock due to salt depletion: comparison of the hemodynamic effects of isotonic saline, of hypertonic saline, and of isotonic glucose solutions. J Clin Invest 1946;25:130–8.

[70] Speedy DB, Noakes TD, Boswell T, et al. Response to a fluid load in athletes with a history of exercise induced hyponatremia. Med Sci Sports Exerc 2001;33(9):1434–42.

[71] Eichner E. Exertional hyponatremia: why so many women? Sports Med Dig 2002;24(5): 54–6.

[72] Davis DP, Videen JS, Marino A, et al. Exercise-associated hyponatremia in marathon runners: a two-year experience. J Emerg Med 2001;21(1):47–57.

[73] Madhusoodanan S, Bogunovic OJ, Moise D, et al. Hyponatraemia associated with psychotropic medications. A review of the literature and spontaneous reports. Adverse Drug React Toxicol Rev 2002;21:17–29.

[74] Sandell RCPM, Noakes TD. factors associated with collapse during and after ultra-marathon footraces: a preliminary study. Phys Sportsmed 1988;16(9):86–94.

ELSEVIER
SAUNDERS

Phys Med Rehabil Clin N Am
16 (2005) 851–858

PHYSICAL MEDICINE
AND REHABILITATION
CLINICS OF
NORTH AMERICA

# Index

*Note:* Page numbers of article titles are in **boldface** type.